FITNESS THERAPY

The complete home reference
to keeping your body strong for life
and dealing with injury

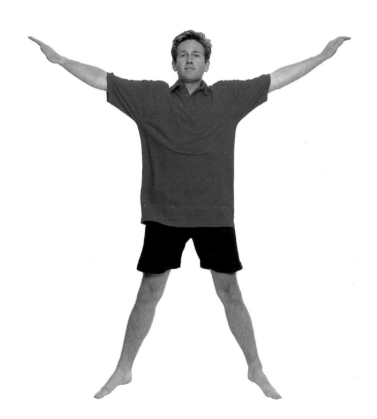

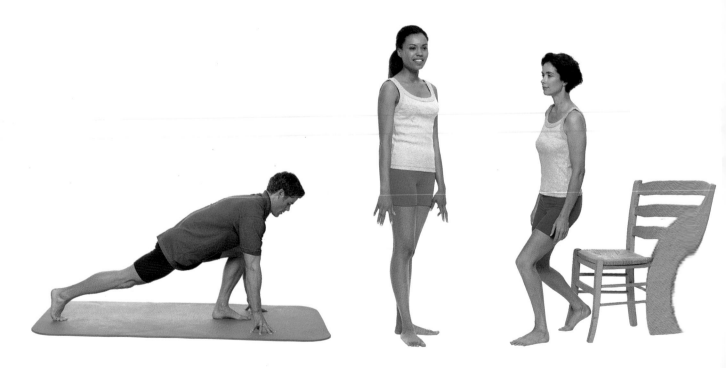

FITNESS THERAPY

The complete home reference
to keeping your body strong for life
and dealing with injury

KATE SHEEHY

MARSHALL PUBLISHING • LONDON

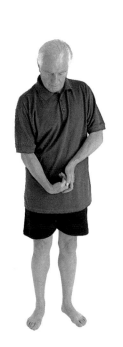
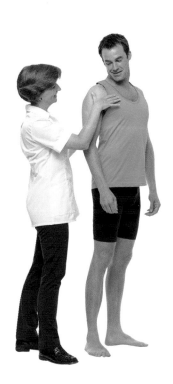
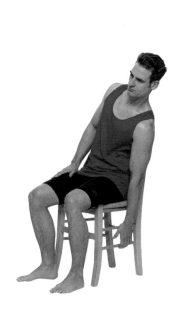

A MARSHALL EDITION
CONCEIVED, EDITED AND DESIGNED BY
MARSHALL EDITIONS LTD
THE ORANGERY
161 NEW BOND STREET
LONDON W1Y 9PA

First published in the UK in 1998 by Marshall Publishing Ltd

ISBN 1-84028-091-3

9 8 7 6 5 4 3 2 1

PROJECT EDITOR CAROLINE TAGGART
MANAGING EDITORS ANNE YELLAND, LINDSAY MCTEAGUE
COPY EDITOR NAOMI PECK
EDITORIAL DIRECTOR SOPHIE COLLINS
ART DIRECTOR SEAN KEOGH
DTP EDITOR LESLEY GILBERT
EDITORIAL COORDINATOR REBECCA CLUNES
DESIGNER VICKY HOLMES
DESIGN ASSISTANT PHILIP LETSU
PRODUCTION NIKKI INGRAM

Originated in Singapore by HBM Print
Printed and bound in Portugal by Printer Portuguesa

Note: Every effort has been taken to ensure that information in
this book is correct. However, this book is not intended to
replace consultation with your doctor, physiotherapist or other
healthcare professional. The author and publisher disclaim any
liability, loss, injury or damage incurred as a consequence,
directly or indirectly, of the use and application of the contents of
this book.

Contents

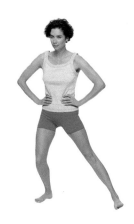

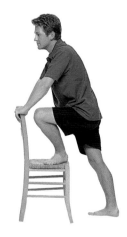

ABOUT PHYSIOTHERAPY

Whether you are young or old, fit or unfit, physiotherapy can help you. Muscles, joints, nerves and ligaments work together in a healthy body, but the balance is easily upset. Physiotherapists treat injury and disease by correcting and improving the body's healing mechanisms, using mobilization and manipulation of joints, guidance on posture, and exercise.

When you consult a physiotherapist, you receive a detailed assessment, individually tailored to your needs. Your physiotherapist will listen to the type of problem you describe and analyse which structures could be affected and how they should be examined. The conclusions from this session form a treatment plan which is used to predict the treatment you might need and the improvement you can expect.

This book is not a substitute for professional treatment by a doctor or physiotherapist. But it includes a carefully worked out programme of exercises that might supplement your treatment. Read the instructions and warnings before you embark on any exercise; and consult a professional if the pain gets worse or if you feel that after one or two weeks of sensible exercise you are not making progress.

Working out a programme of exercises requires you to use your common sense and listen to the messages your body is giving you. Follow these simple guidelines and you will help your body to heal itself, without causing any further injury.

EQUIPMENT

Some basic equipment is needed for a few of the exercises in this book. Small weights weighing 250 g or 500 g (9 oz or 18 oz) are available from sports shops. Some are held in your hand, others take the form of wrist bands.

Beginner

Elastic exercise bands – marketed under the brand names Cliniband or Theraband – are available at some sports shops or from your physiotherapist. They come on a roll so that you can cut a length that suits you and the specific exercise (you will obviously need less if you are wrapping the band round your fingers than if you are standing with it passed under your foot). They are like extra wide elastic bands which allow you to work against gently controlled resistance. They also come in different strengths, providing varying degrees of resistance.

Intermediate

Advanced

CAUTION

Certain types of injury and arthritis can cause a great deal of joint swelling (inflammation). The knee, for instance, can become very inflamed. When this happens it looks red and feels hot to the touch, the skin is taut and any movement is sore. At this stage it is unwise to do any exercise: firstly it will be too painful and secondly the pain and swelling will prevent your muscles from working normally – so the exercises do not achieve their aim. It is best to consult your doctor or physiotherapist about how to tackle this sort of inflammation and follow their advice about when to start exercising.

WORKING OUT YOUR OWN TREATMENT PROGRAMME

● **The book is divided into nine principal chapters,** each dedicated to a different part of the body. Choose only the chapter(s) that are appropriate to you.

● **At the beginning of each chapter is a chart showing the exercises classified into three categories –** mobility, flexibility, and strength and stability – and three levels of difficulty – beginner, intermediate and advanced. Start at the beginners' level, following the instructions given at the head of each chart.

● **Mobility exercises are best done as gentle, nudging actions to coax a little more movement from the joint and to encourage lubrication over the joint surfaces.** As you do the exercises you should feel initial resistance followed by more "give" in the joint. Sometimes you will feel some soreness around the joint as you do the exercise, but this should settle soon after you stop.

● **Flexibility exercises depend more on your sustaining a position** (although at first this may be only a few seconds) to achieve a stretch, then repeating once or twice at the beginners' level and gradually increasing the number of repeats up to four or five.

● **Strength and stability exercises require repetition to achieve their aim.** Muscles respond to demand, so you need to repeat the exercises until your muscles feel tired (or fatigued). At this point the muscles will sometimes "shudder" or you may feel a twinge of cramp. This means that you are working the muscle effectively; more serious cramp makes you stop working.

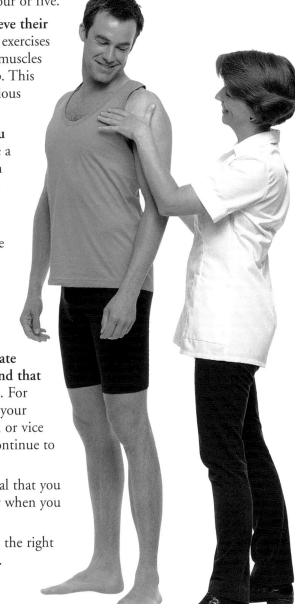

● **You must judge for yourself how the exercises feel as you do them.** They should not cause too much discomfort. Take a movement to the point of pain, but not through it. Pain can be a signal from your body that you are pushing it too hard.

● **Try to do your exercises every day and at the same time each day.** Be realistic: tell yourself you are going to exercise for 10 minutes a day – then you can be sure you will achieve your target. Later you may feel able to move up to 10 minutes twice a day.

● **Start very gently.** If you have a serious injury, you may find that all the exercises are difficult or painful. In this case, seek guidance from your doctor or physiotherapist.

● **When you progress from the beginners' to the intermediate level or from intermediate to advanced, you are likely to find that you have problems with a similar type of exercise as before.** For example, you may find the exercises involving straightening your knee more difficult than those which require you to bend it, or vice versa. This is perfectly normal and shows that you should continue to concentrate on that area.

● **Be patient.** Everybody heals at a different rate and it is vital that you work at a level that is comfortable for you and progress only when you feel ready.

● **Age is not a barrier to exercise** – you just need to work at the right level and feel comfortable with the exercises as you do them.

HOW TO USE THIS BOOK

Each of the first nine chapters of this book deals with a specific part of the body which might benefit from physiotherapy after an injury, and provides a graduated course of exercises with step-by-step instructions. The tenth and final chapter is about injuries that might occur as a result of exercise and explains how best to avoid these.

HOW TO BEGIN

Before starting any exercise, read "About Physiotherapy" (pages 6–7) and the introduction to the relevant chapter carefully, and follow the instructions. The first two pages outline the sort of injury or complaint that may affect this part of the body. They also classify the exercises according to type and level of difficulty and explain how to identify the exercises that are of most benefit to your particular problem.

Opening symbol follows the colour coding of the rest of the chapter.

Explanatory text describes likely causes of problems in this area.

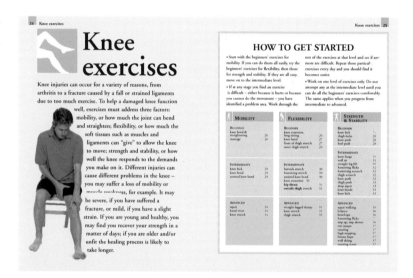

Text explains how to plan your exercise programme.

Beginners' exercises.

Intermediate exercises.

Advanced exercises.

SYMBOLS AND COLOURS

The exercises are divided into three levels of difficulty – beginners', intermediate and advanced – and three types – mobility, flexibility, and strength and stability. The specific applications of these three categories are explained on page 7. Throughout the book, the symbols illustrated here are used to designate the three different types of exercise.

The levels of difficulty are identified by colour coding of the models' clothing. For the beginners' exercises, their shirts or shorts are blue; for the intermediate ones, they are turquoise; and for the advanced ones, red.

For easy identification when flipping through the book, each chapter is also colour coded so that the background to the introduction and the panels with the exercise names, and page numbers are the same colour.

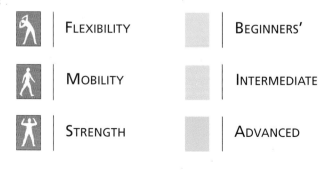

FLEXIBILITY	BEGINNERS'
MOBILITY	INTERMEDIATE
STRENGTH	ADVANCED

THE EXERCISE PAGES

These form the core of the book, with some 30 to 50 exercises for each part of the body. Each exercise is clearly explained, with step by step instructions enhanced by colour photography showing precisely what you are supposed to do.

Exercises are divided into three levels – beginners', intermediate and advanced – with a paragraph at the start of each section reinforcing the advice and cautions about progress given at the start of the chapter.

THE GYM PAGES

The last chapter in the book is devoted to one of the most common causes of damage to the joints – the wrong kind of exercise. If you use gym equipment incorrectly, you will do yourself more harm than good. The chapter emphasises the importance of precision when working out on gym machines in order to avoid injury. Trunk stability is crucial to safe gym work, as is proximal stability – that is, strong and stable shoulders and hips. Similarly, if you lack full flexibility in your limbs, you risk injury when you work with weights in the gym.

Colour coding makes it easy to identify each chapter at a glance.

Introductory text helps you work out your own routine.

Step by step photographs enhance the instructions.

Symbols indicate the type of exercise.

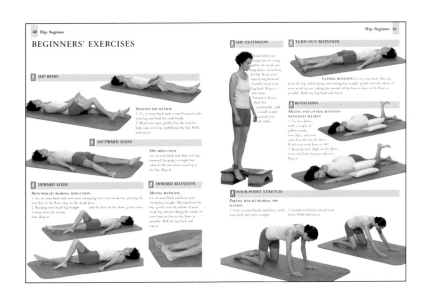

Colour coding continues in exercise names.

Popular name makes each exercise approachable.

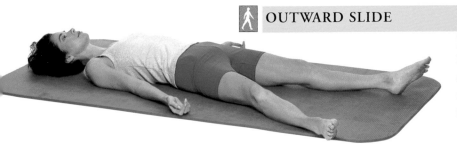

![symbol] OUTWARD SLIDE

HIP ABDUCTION
Lie on your back and slide your leg outward, keeping it straight but relaxed. Do not rotate your leg at the hip. Repeat.

Technical name gives medical description of the benefit of an exercise.

Arrows show the direction of subtle movements.

Foot & Ankle Exercises

The most common ankle injury is a sprain or strain, which occurs when the fibres of the ligament (which run from bone to bone and hold the side of the joint together) get overstretched. Even after the tissues have apparently healed, the ankle may not be fully retrained in terms of balance. The ligaments are packed with nerve receptors which sense position. This information is transmitted to the brain, and messages are sent back down again to keep us balanced. If this function is not re-educated, the foot and ankle are not ready to respond to uneven surfaces or difficult terrain and the previously damaged ligament will be vulnerable.

If you are recovering from an ankle injury, make sure you are really competent with the balance exercises in this chapter as well as those for mobility and flexibility – this will give you the best chance of avoiding another injury.

HOW TO GET STARTED

• Start with the beginners' exercises for mobility. If you can do them all easily, try the beginners' exercises for flexibility, then those for strength and stability. If they are all easy, move on to the intermediate level.

• If at any stage you find an exercise is difficult – either because it hurts or because you cannot do the movement – you have identified a problem area. Work through the rest of the exercises at that level and see if any more are difficult. Repeat those particular exercises every day and you should find they become easier.

• Work on one level of exercises only. Do not attempt any at the intermediate level until you can do all the beginners' exercises comfortably. The same applies when you progress from the intermediate level to the advanced.

MOBILITY

BEGINNER
Ankle stretches	12
Foot turn-in	12
Foot turn-out	12
Foot & toe stretch	13
Ankle stretch	13
Foot turn-out	13
Foot turn-in	13

INTERMEDIATE
Ankle turn-out & turn-in	16
Ankle stretches	16
Foot turn-out & turn-in	17
Toe mobility	17

ADVANCED
Kneeling	20
Kneeling with overpressure	20
Squatting	20
Foot stretch	21

FLEXIBILITY

BEGINNER
Lower leg mobility	14
Ankle mobility	14
Mid-foot & toe flexibility	14
Foot stretch	15
Ankle stretch	15

INTERMEDIATE
Calf stretches	18
Achilles stretch	18
Ankle stretch	18

ADVANCED
Ankle stretch	20
Calf stretch	21
Achilles stretch	21

STRENGTH & STABILITY

BEGINNER
Toe flexions	15
Ankle flexions	15

INTERMEDIATE
Weight transference	19
Toe agility	19
Heel raises	19
Toe tapping	19
Balance	19

ADVANCED
Toe agility	21
Step-ups	22
Walking	22
Heel raises	23
Balance	23
Running	23
Arch raises	23

BEGINNERS' EXERCISES

These exercises aim to restore some mobility in the foot and ankle, while encouraging muscle control and increasing flexibility in the soft tissues. Don't worry if you can't take the movements very far or hold them for more than a few seconds. Do only what feels comfortable.

ANKLE STRETCH

PLANTAR FLEXION

Sit with your legs straight out in front of you. Put your hands on the floor by your sides for support if necessary. You could also lie on the floor with your legs straight.

Point your whole foot and ankle and feel a gentle stretch in your ankle and the top of your foot. Hold, relax and repeat.

FOOT TURN-IN

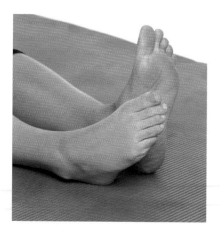

INVERSION

Starting in the same position as above, turn your whole foot and ankle inward, toward your mid-line. You should feel a gentle stretch on the outside of your calf and ankle. Hold, relax and repeat.

ANKLE STRETCH

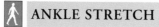

DORSI FLEXION

Starting in the same position as above, use the muscles in your foot and lower leg to flex your whole foot and ankle toward your body. You should feel a gentle stretch at the back of your calf and ankle. Hold, relax and repeat.

FOOT TURN-OUT

EVERSION

Starting in the same position as above, turn your whole foot and ankle outward, away from your mid-line, so that you feel a gentle stretch on the inside of your calf and ankle. Hold, relax and repeat.

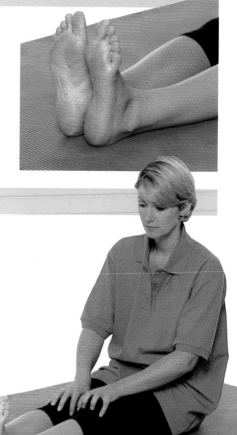

🚶 FOOT & TOE STRETCH

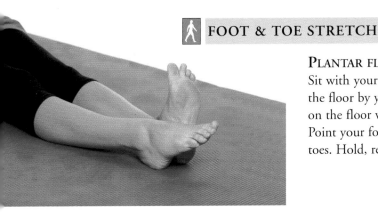

PLANTAR FLEXION

Sit with your legs straight out in front of you. Put your hands on the floor by your sides for support if necessary. You could also lie on the floor with your legs straight.

Point your foot and ankle, concentrating on the mid-foot and toes. Hold, relax and repeat.

🚶 ANKLE STRETCH

DORSI FLEXION

Starting in the same position as above, use the muscles of your foot and lower leg to draw your foot and ankle up toward your body, concentrating on the mid-foot and toes. Hold, relax and repeat.

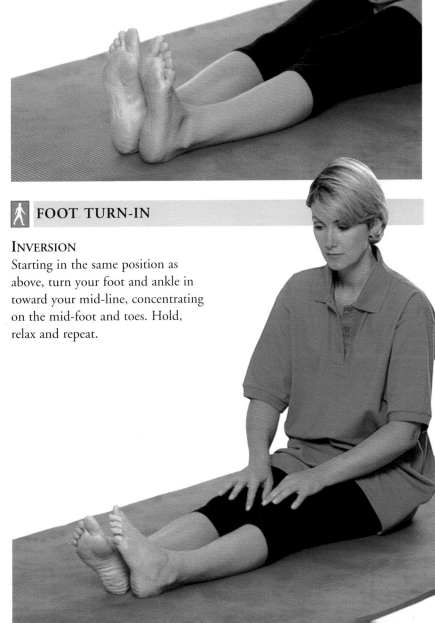

🚶 FOOT TURN-OUT

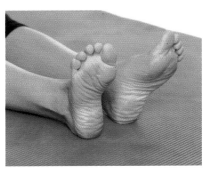

EVERSION

Starting in the same position as above, turn your foot and ankle outward, away from your mid-line, concentrating on the mid-foot and toes. Hold, relax and repeat.

🚶 FOOT TURN-IN

INVERSION

Starting in the same position as above, turn your foot and ankle in toward your mid-line, concentrating on the mid-foot and toes. Hold, relax and repeat.

LOWER LEG MOBILITY

ANTERIOR LOWER LIMB STRETCH

Lie face down on the floor, with your head resting on your crossed forearms. Bend your leg at the knee, taking your weak foot toward your buttock as far as is comfortable and pointing your toes. Hold, relax and repeat.

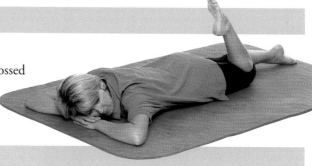

 ANKLE MOBILITY

ANKLE PLANTAR & DORSI FLEXION, INVERSION & EVERSION

Sit on the floor with your strong leg straight out in front of you and your weak leg bent so that the ankle rests on the opposite thigh, just above the knee.

1 Grasp your ankle with the hand on your weak side, pressing the thumb against your heel bone and the fingers on the top of your ankle. Use your other hand to pull your foot toward you. Relax and repeat.

2 Cup your heel with the hand on your strong side and push away from your body, grasping the sole with your other hand and pulling the foot up toward you. Relax and repeat.

3 Press the side of your heel bone with the thumb of the hand on your strong side, using the fingers to turn the middle of the foot. With the fingers of the hand on your weak side, grasp your foot just below the toes and rotate it in. Relax and repeat.

4 Grasp your foot with both hands, the hand on your strong side holding the heel and the other hand holding the ball of the foot. Use the fingers of both hands to twist your foot out. Relax and repeat.

1

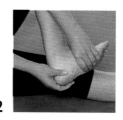 **2** 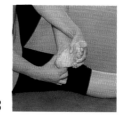 **3** 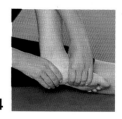 **4**

 MID-FOOT AND TOE FLEXIBILITY

Start in the same position as for the Ankle Mobility exercise above.

1 Clasp both hands over your toes and gently pull them downward. Relax and repeat.

2 Push the thumb of your other hand into the middle of the top of your foot, grasping the underside with your fingers. Using the hand on your weak side, pull your toes toward your body, while at the same time pushing them away with your thumb. Relax and repeat.

3 Grasp the top of your foot in both hands with both thumbs on the sole. Twist your foot away from you, turning the sole in toward your body. Relax and repeat. Then grasp the sole of your foot with both hands and rotate it away from your body. Relax and repeat.

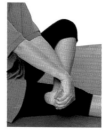 **1** 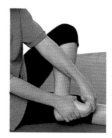 **2** 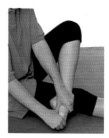 **3**

FOOT STRETCH

ASSISTED DORSI FLEXION
Sit on the floor with your legs straight out in front of you. Loop a towel round your weak foot. Keeping your heel on the floor and pulling with both hands, use the towel to draw the mid-foot and toes toward your body. Hold for a few seconds. Keep your other leg relaxed. Repeat.

ANKLE STRETCH

ANKLE FLEXION
Sit with your legs straight out in front of you. Point your foot down and then bring it toward you as far as is comfortable. Hold, relax and repeat.

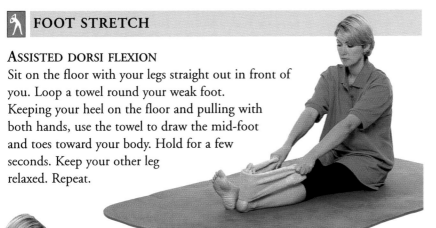

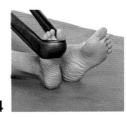

1

 ## TOE FLEXIONS

DORSI & PLANTAR FLEXION, INVERSION & EVERSION
Sitting with your legs out in front of you, wrap an elastic exercise band round your foot and hold the ends firmly. Repeat the exercises on page 12, flexing your foot and ankle toward you (1), pointing them away (2), turning them in (3) and out (4). Your foot and ankle will work against the resistance of the band. Remember to point your toes. Repeat until fatigued.

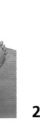

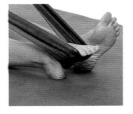
2

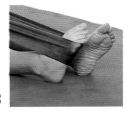
3

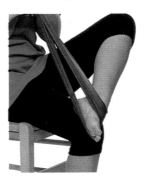
4

ANKLE FLEXIONS

1

Sit on an upright chair with the arm on your strong side hooked over the back of the chair to stop it from moving. Rest your weak ankle on your other thigh just above the knee.
1 Loop the elastic exercise band over the middle of your foot, holding both ends on the strong side of your body. Flex your toes and pull your foot up toward you, working against the band.
2 Move the band to your ankle and repeat the same movement.
3 Holding the band on your other side with your other hand, point your toes downward.
4 Return the band to the middle of your foot and repeat the same movement.

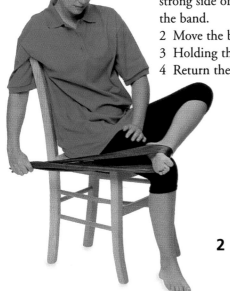

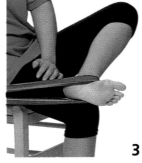
2

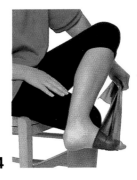
3

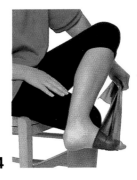
4

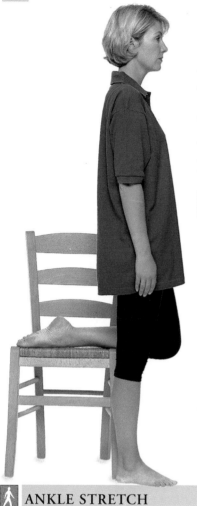

INTERMEDIATE EXERCISES

Move on to these exercises only when you are comfortable with the beginners' ones. The affected joint should feel stronger, and you should have more flexibility and range of movement in the affected areas. You should be able to hold positions a little longer, and repeat about 6 to 8 times.

ANKLE TURN-OUT & TURN-IN

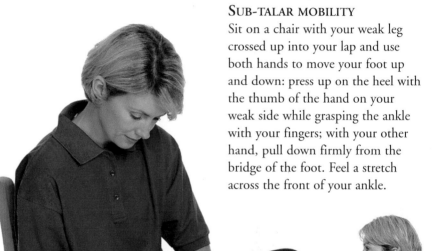

SUB-TALAR MOBILITY

Sit on a chair with your weak leg crossed up into your lap and use both hands to move your foot up and down: press up on the heel with the thumb of the hand on your weak side while grasping the ankle with your fingers; with your other hand, pull down firmly from the bridge of the foot. Feel a stretch across the front of your ankle.

ANKLE STRETCH

PLANTAR FLEXION
Stand next to a chair with your weak knee bent so that your shin and foot rest on the seat. Point your toes, hold, relax and repeat.

ANKLE STRETCH

DORSI FLEXION
Stand facing a chair. Put the toes and front of your weak foot on the chair but let the heel drop down. Hold this position, aiming for a gentle stretch along the Achilles tendon at the back of the heel.

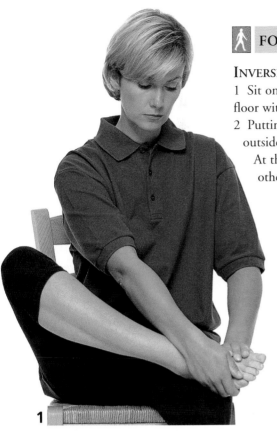

FOOT TURN-OUT & TURN-IN

INVERSION & EVERSION

1 Sit on a chair with your weak leg crossed up into your lap (or sit on the floor with your legs crossed).

2 Putting the thumb of the hand on your weak side on your heel, grip the outside of your foot with your fingers and pull the foot gently toward you. At the same time, push gently down on the top of your foot with your other hand. You should feel the effect across the top of your foot.

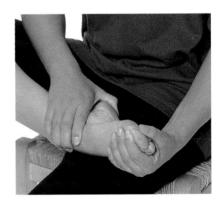

1

2

TOE MOBILITY

PLANTAR & DORSI FLEXION & ABDUCTION

1 Start in the same position as above. Hold your ankle with the hand on your weak side, and gently pull your toes toward you with your other hand.

2 Then gently push your toes away from you.

3 Interlock your fingers with your toes, using the fingers to push the toes apart. You should feel a stretch between the toes.

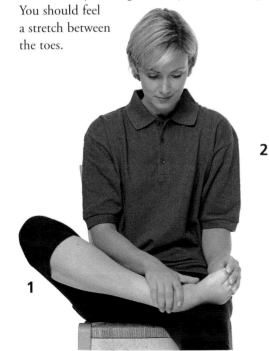

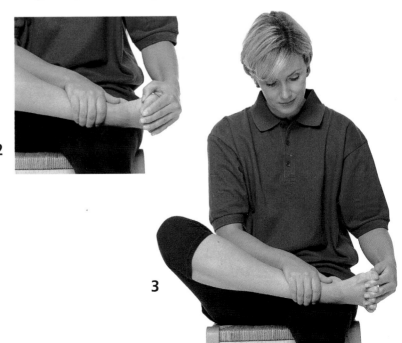

1

2

3

CALF STRETCH

GASTROCNEMIUS ACHILLES LENGTH

Stand leaning against a wall, hands resting on it, with your weak leg behind your strong one, about one hip's width away. Let your strong leg take more than half your weight. Keep the back knee straight and lean into the wall so that you can feel a stretch in your calf. Hold.

ACHILLES STRETCH

ACHILLES LENGTH

1 Stand next to a chair with the ball of your weak foot resting on a step or thick book.
2 Lean on the back of the chair for support. Lift your strong foot off the floor, letting the heel of your weak foot drop down so that you feel a stretch in the Achilles tendon at the back of the heel.
Hold the position, relax and repeat.

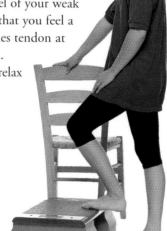

1

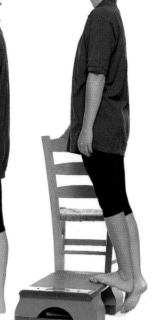

2

CALF STRETCH

SOLEUS LENGTH

Stand leaning against a wall, hands resting on it, with your weak leg positioned behind your strong one, about one hip's width away. Your strong leg takes more of your weight; bend your back knee so that you can feel a stretch in your lower calf. Hold.

ANKLE STRETCH

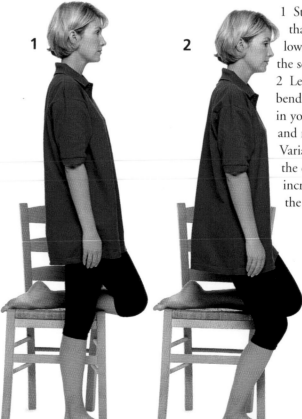

1

2

1 Stand next to a chair, so that your weak foot and lower leg are resting on the seat. Point your toes.
2 Let your strong knee bend to increase the stretch in your foot. Hold, relax and repeat.
Variation: turn the foot on the chair in and out to increase the flexibility in the ankle.

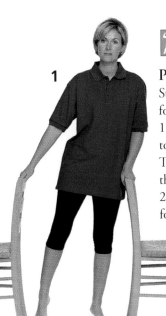

1

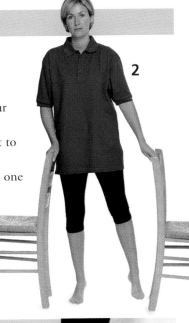

2

WEIGHT TRANSFERENCE

PARTIAL WEIGHT-BEARING MOBILITY

Stand between two chairs, or lean against a wall or table for support.

1 Keeping your feet about a hip's width apart, stand on your toes and transfer weight from one foot to the other. Repeat. Then stand on your heels and transfer weight from one foot to the other. Repeat.

2 Stand on the inside of your feet and transfer weight from one foot to the other. Repeat. Then stand on the outside of your feet and transfer weight from one foot to the other. Repeat.

TOE AGILITY

LUMBRICALS

Sit on a chair with a towel on the floor under your toes and stretched out away from your foot. Keeping your foot flat, use your toes to drag the towel back toward your foot, so that the towel bunches up. Repeat until fatigued.

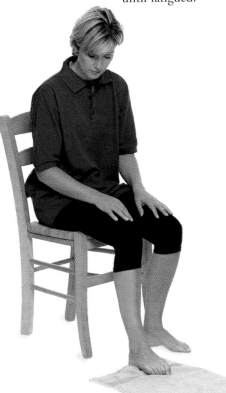

HEEL RAISES

SOLEUS & GASTROCNEMIUS

Stand leaning against a wall or table for support. Keeping your feet quite close together, lift both heels off the floor. Repeat. This exercise strengthens the calf muscles.

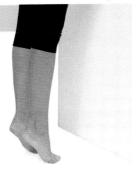

TOE TAPPING

ANTERIOR TIBIALS

Sit on a chair and tap your weak foot. Repeat until fatigued. This strengthens the muscles at the front of the lower leg. Variations: turn the foot in or out slightly before you start.

BALANCE

PROPRIOCEPTION

Stand between two chairs and lean lightly on them (use your fingertips only – do not grip the chairs). Lift your strong leg and balance on the weak one only. Take care not to roll the supporting foot. Repeat and aim to stand perfectly still.

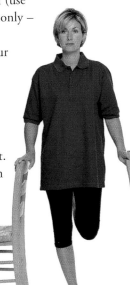

KNEELING

PLANTAR FLEXION OVERPRESSURE

Kneel, sitting on your heels with your back straight and your hands on your thighs. Hold. This increases mobility in the front of the ankle joint, and between the heel and the foot. Variations: turn your foot in more; turn it out more.

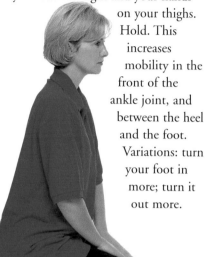

ADVANCED EXERCISES

By the time you progress to this stage you should be able to achieve almost the normal range of movement in the affected joints and cope with more sustained holds and strong stretches. Repeat all the exercises until fatigued.

KNEELING WITH OVERPRESSURE

SUB-TALAR OVERPRESSURE

Kneel on the floor, sitting back on your heels with your back straight. Use your hands to press forward on your heels to extend the stretch. Hold.

SQUATTING

FULL WEIGHT-BEARING MOBILITY

1 With your back straight and head up, squat with your heels. Hold.
2 Lower your heels to the floor, stretching your arms out in front to help you balance if necessary. Hold.

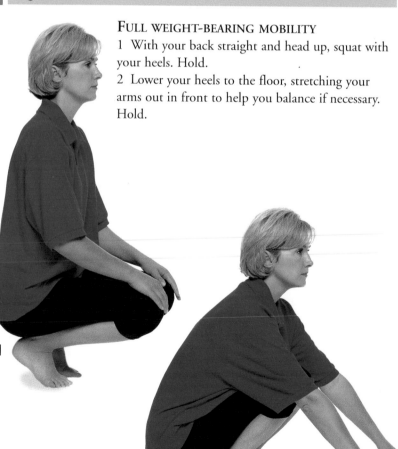

1

2

ANKLE STRETCH

ANTERIOR LOWER LIMB LENGTH

Standing, bend your leg so that your weak foot is raised toward your buttock. Point your toes and hold them in your hand to increase the stretch in your ankle. Hold.

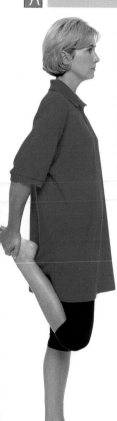

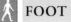 ## CALF STRETCH

SOLEUS LENGTH

Stand with your strong leg in front of your weak one, bend the weak knee slightly and lean forward, with most of your weight on your strong leg. Hold. Variation: repeat the exercise keeping your weak knee straight.

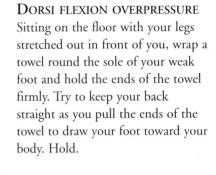

FOOT STRETCH

DORSI FLEXION OVERPRESSURE

Sitting on the floor with your legs stretched out in front of you, wrap a towel round the sole of your weak foot and hold the ends of the towel firmly. Try to keep your back straight as you pull the ends of the towel to draw your foot toward your body. Hold.

 ## ACHILLES STRETCH

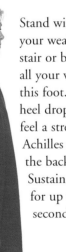

Stand with the ball of your weak foot on a stair or block, with all your weight on this foot. Let your heel drop down and feel a stretch in the Achilles tendon at the back of the heel. Sustain the position for up to 15 seconds.

TOE AGILITY

PROPRIOCEPTION

Sit on a chair that is high enough for your feet to rest comfortably on the floor. Practise picking up objects such as a ball of cotton wool, a pen or a bunch of keys with your toes, curling your toes under your foot to hold the object in place. Hold.

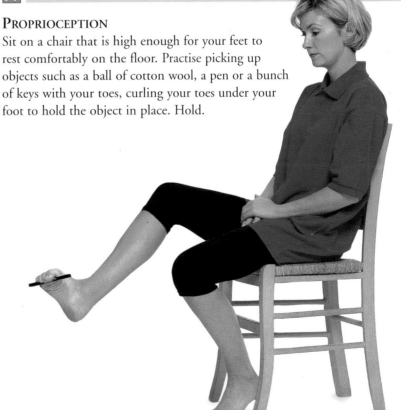

STEP-UPS

Calf power

1 Stand facing a step or block. Step up with your weak leg, then your strong one, so that both feet are on the block. Step down with your weak leg, then your strong one. Repeat. Start by doing the exercise slowly, gradually increasing your speed as you feel more able. This helps to build up strength in your calves.

2 Variation: lead with the other leg so that you take your weight on your weak leg as you step down with your strong one.

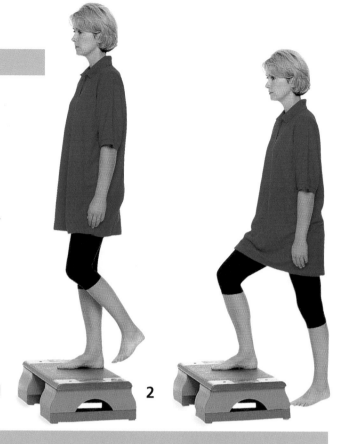

1

2

 WALKING

Proprioception & strength

Walk across the room on your toes (1), on your heels (2), on the outside of your feet (3) and on the inside of your feet (4). Look at your feet to help with balance. Repeat until fatigued. Concentrate on the aspects of this exercise which feel most awkward.

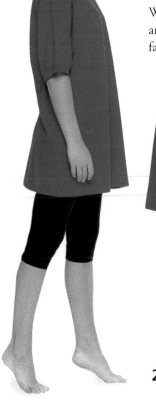

1

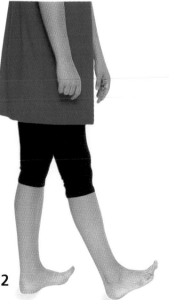

2

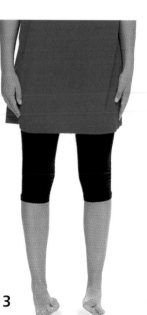

3

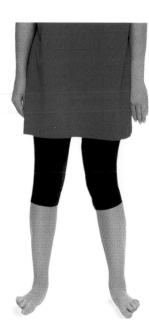

4

HEEL RAISES

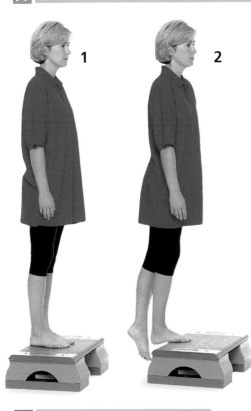

1 2 3

PLANTAR FLEXION POWER

1 Stand on a block or step.

2 Step back slightly so that your strong leg hangs freely and the heel of your weak foot drops below the level of the step.

3 Raise your heel to the level of the step, then go up on your toes. Use your arms to balance, or put the step next to a wall or chair for support. Repeat. This exercise is good for strengthening the calf muscles.

BALANCE

PROPRIOCEPTION

To improve balance, stand on your weak leg with the knee slightly bent. Bend your strong knee and raise your foot off the ground. Swing your torso round toward your strong side, then back. Try to keep your eyes closed.

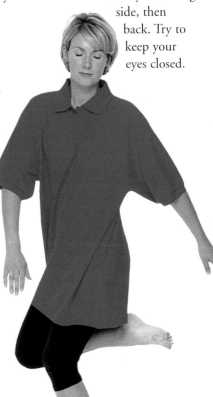

RUNNING

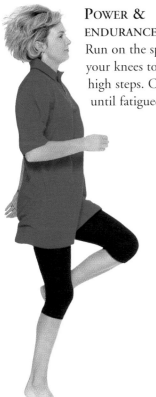

POWER & ENDURANCE

Run on the spot, lifting your knees to make high steps. Continue until fatigued.

ARCH RAISES

LUMBRICALS

Standing on your weak leg, spread your toes and grip the floor with your toes to raise the transverse arch across the base of your toe. At the same time, raise the inside arch along the length of your foot. Keep your heel on the floor. Repeat.

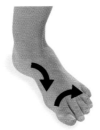

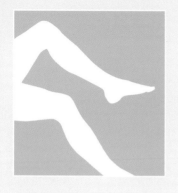

Knee Exercises

Knee injuries can occur for a variety of reasons, from arthritis to a fracture caused by a fall to strained ligaments due to too much exercise. To help a damaged knee function well, exercises must address three factors: mobility, or how much the joint can bend and straighten; flexibility, or how much the soft tissues such as muscles and ligaments can "give" to allow the knee to move; strength and stability, or how well the knee responds to the demands you make on it. Different injuries can cause different problems in the knee – you may suffer a loss of mobility or muscle weakness, for example. It may be severe – if you have suffered a fracture – or mild – if you have a slight strain. If you are young and healthy, you may find you recover your strength in a matter of days; if you are older and/or unfit the healing process is likely to take longer.

HOW TO GET STARTED

• Start with the beginners' exercises for mobility. If you can do them all easily, try the beginners' exercises for flexibility, then those for strength and stability. If they are all easy, move on to the intermediate level.

• If at any stage you find an exercise is difficult – either because it hurts or because you cannot do the movement – you have identified a problem area. Work through the rest of the exercises at that level and see if any more are difficult. Repeat those particular exercises every day and you should find they become easier.

• Work on one level of exercises only. Do not attempt any at the intermediate level until you can do all the beginners' exercises comfortably. The same applies when you progress from the intermediate to the advanced level.

MOBILITY

BEGINNER
Knee bend & straightening	26

INTERMEDIATE
Knee lock	29
Knee bend	29
Assisted knee bend	29

ADVANCED
Squat	34
Kneel twist	34
Knee stretch	34

FLEXIBILITY

BEGINNER
Massage	26
Upper thigh stretch	26
Knee bend	27
Front of thigh stretch	27
Outer thigh stretch	27

INTERMEDIATE
Buttock stretch	30
Hamstring stretch	30
Assisted knee bend	30
Knee extension	30
Hip thrust	31
Outside thigh stretch	31

ADVANCED
Straight-legged slump	35
Knee stretch	35
Thigh stretch	35

STRENGTH & STABILITY

BEGINNER
Knee lock	28
Thigh lock	28
Knee push	28
Knee bends	28
Heel push	28

INTERMEDIATE
Knee lunge	31
Wall sit	31
Straight leg lift	31
Hamstring flicks	32
Hamstring scrunch	32
Thigh scrunch	32
Knee push	32
Thigh push	33
Deep squat	33
Knee bends	33
Knee lock	33

ADVANCED
Squat walking	35
Balance	36
Kneel-ups	36
Hamstring flicks	36
Step-ups, step-downs	36
Star jumps	37
Running	37
High stepping	37
Bunny hops	37
Wall skiing	37
Running starts	37

BEGINNERS' EXERCISES

These exercises aim to introduce mobility, flexbility and strength to the knee joint and surrounding soft tissue. As with all the beginners' exercises in this book, you should repeat them only as often as is comfortable – at this stage it is important not to overwork or strain the knee. Don't worry if you cannot take the movement very far or do it more than a couple of times: it will become easier as you work at it patiently.

 KNEE BEND & STRAIGHTENING

Lie on your back with your legs straight. Put a rolled-up towel under your weak knee if this is more comfortable. Gently bend the knee and straighten it again, emphasizing the "rest phase" at the end of the movement. Repeat. This exercise allows gravity to enhance the stretch on the knee.

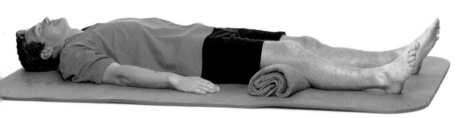

 UPPER THIGH STRETCH

Sit on the floor with your legs stretched out in front of you. Place a small pillow or a couple of towels under the ankle on your weak side to extend the knee. Put your hands on the floor to support your upper body. Hold the position for up to 5 minutes, letting your knee stretch. Gently bend the knee, then hold the stretch again.

MASSAGE

Sit on a chair with your weak leg slightly bent. Massage the area around the kneecap. You should feel the tissues loosen under your fingers.

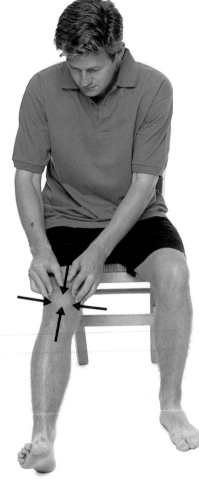

KNEE BEND

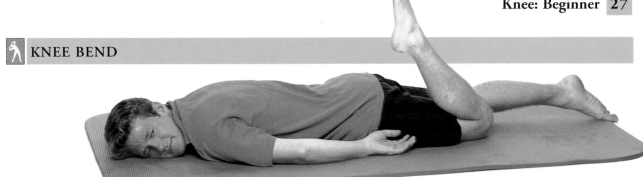

Lie on your front with your head to one side and your arms at your sides. Keep your strong leg and foot relaxed and flat on the floor. Without moving your hips, bend your weak knee and take your leg up as close to your buttock as is comfortable. Hold. Relax, taking your foot back down to the floor, then repeat. This improves the mobility of the knee joint and allows the muscles on the front of the thigh to lengthen.

FRONT OF THIGH STRETCH

Lie on your back with your strong leg bent up toward your chest. Keeping your other leg and knee extended and your toes and feet relaxed, hug the raised knee with your arms and let your weak leg relax down. You should feel a stretch in the front of your weak thigh and up into your hip.

OUTER THIGH STRETCH

Lie on your strong side, with a pillow between your knees and another under your head. This position will gently stretch the outer thigh on your weak leg. Hold for up to 5 minutes.

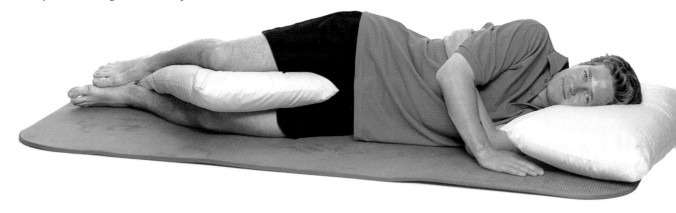

KNEE LOCK

QUADRICEPS CONTROL

Sit on a chair with your weak leg stretched out in front of you but not tense. Hold the inside edge of your kneecap, keeping it still, and tighten your front thigh muscles so that your kneecap pushes against your thumb. Hold, relax and repeat.

THIGH LOCK

STATIC QUADRICEPS

Sit on the floor with your legs stretched out in front of you and your hands on the floor to help you to sit upright. Tighten the muscles at the front of your thigh and pull your toes up toward you as far as is comfortable. Hold, relax and repeat.

KNEE PUSH

STATIC QUADRICEPS

Lie on your front with your head to one side. Hook your strong foot over your weak ankle and gently push your weak leg toward the strong one. At the same time, keep your strong leg tense and resist the movement so that both legs remain in the same position. Hold, relax and repeat.

KNEE BENDS

PARTIAL WEIGHT-BEARING KNEE FLEXION

Stand between two chairs, with your hands on the backs for support. Bend your elbows to relax your shoulders and allow your weight to drop as you bend your knees. Repeat 2 to 3 times.

HEEL PUSH

HAMSTRING & GLUTEAL CONTROL

Lie on your front with your arms by your sides and your head relaxed and to one side. With your knees apart, bend them so that your feet are pointing up in the air, then push your heels together. Hold, relax and repeat.

THIGH LOCK

GLUTEALS, HAMSTRINGS & ADDUCTORS

Sit on a table, using your hands to help you balance. Bend your knees to an angle of 45 degrees and place the heel of your strong foot against the instep of your weak one, with your toes pointing out. Push your heel and instep together, using the same force from each side. Relax and repeat.

INTERMEDIATE EXERCISES

Once you are comfortable with the beginners' exercises, move on to this section. You should find that you have a greater range of movement and are able to continue the exercises longer without becoming fatigued. In many cases you will feel a gentle stretch, but remember not to push yourself so far that it becomes painful.

 ## KNEE LOCK

KNEE EXTENSION

Sit on the floor with your legs out in front of you. Support the heel on your weak side with one or two towels so that it is higher than the knee. Keeping the other leg relaxed, extend your leg and straighten the knee. Gently bounce the knee up and down to loosen the joint and then sustain the extension. Repeat.

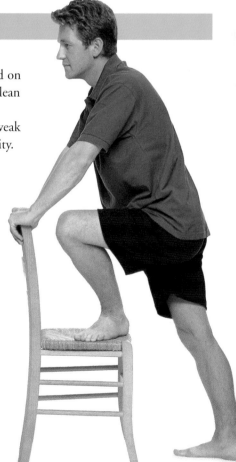

 ## KNEE BEND

PARTIAL WEIGHT-BEARING KNEE BEND

Standing, bend your weak knee and place your foot on the seat of a chair. Hold on to the chair back. Keeping your other leg straight and the foot facing forward, lean into the chair, bending your knee further. Hold, relax and repeat.
Variations: turn your weak foot out, lean forward, hold and repeat; turn your weak foot in, lean forward, hold and repeat. This exercise increases knee-bend mobility.

ASSISTED KNEE BEND

KNEE FLEXION

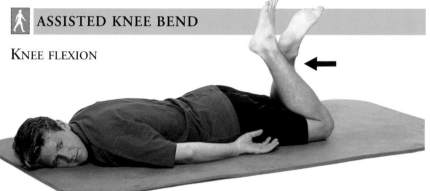

Lie on your front with your head to one side and your arms at your sides. Bend your knees, then cross the foot of your strong leg over the shin of your weak one. Press the strong foot gently against the weak leg, pushing it toward your buttock with small repetitive movements, then hold. Relax and repeat.

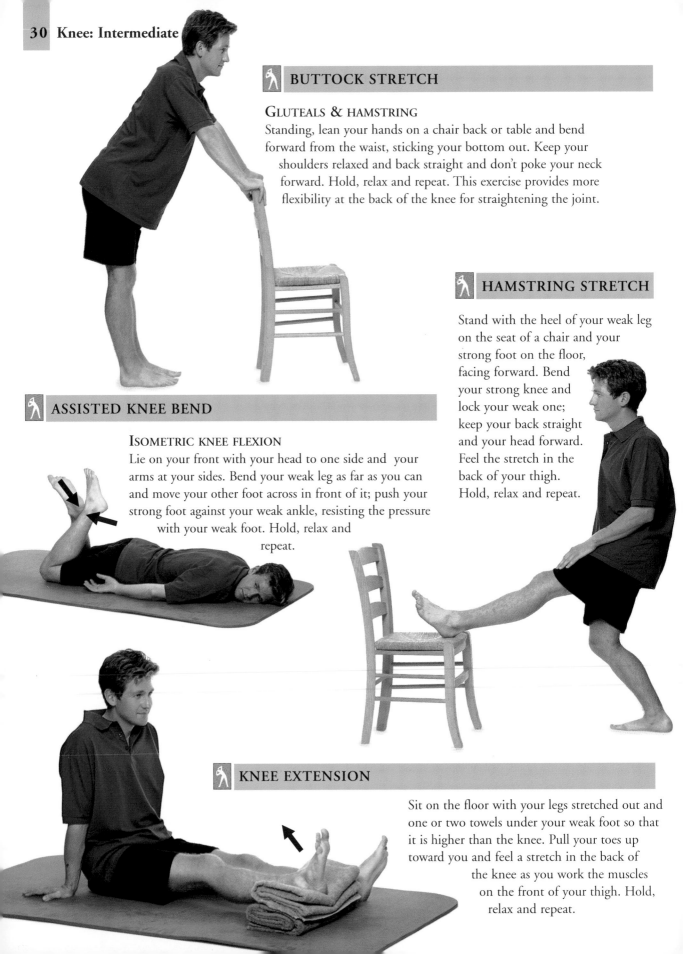

BUTTOCK STRETCH

GLUTEALS & HAMSTRING

Standing, lean your hands on a chair back or table and bend forward from the waist, sticking your bottom out. Keep your shoulders relaxed and back straight and don't poke your neck forward. Hold, relax and repeat. This exercise provides more flexibility at the back of the knee for straightening the joint.

HAMSTRING STRETCH

Stand with the heel of your weak leg on the seat of a chair and your strong foot on the floor, facing forward. Bend your strong knee and lock your weak one; keep your back straight and your head forward. Feel the stretch in the back of your thigh. Hold, relax and repeat.

ASSISTED KNEE BEND

ISOMETRIC KNEE FLEXION

Lie on your front with your head to one side and your arms at your sides. Bend your weak leg as far as you can and move your other foot across in front of it; push your strong foot against your weak ankle, resisting the pressure with your weak foot. Hold, relax and repeat.

KNEE EXTENSION

Sit on the floor with your legs stretched out and one or two towels under your weak foot so that it is higher than the knee. Pull your toes up toward you and feel a stretch in the back of the knee as you work the muscles on the front of your thigh. Hold, relax and repeat.

HIP THRUST

Stand with your knee bent at a 90-degree angle and your lower leg resting on a chair, with the ankle supported. Pull your stomach up and in, squeeze your buttocks and thrust your hips forward. Hold, relax and repeat. This increases

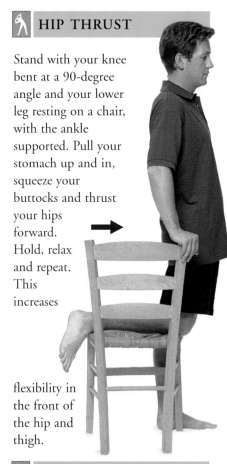

flexibility in the front of the hip and thigh.

KNEE LUNGE

STRENGTHENING QUADRICEPS & HAMSTRINGS
Stand between two chairs, with your weak leg in front of your strong one. Bend your arms and gently lunge forward, bending both knees. Relax and repeat.

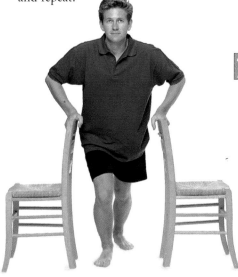

OUTSIDE THIGH STRETCH

ILIOTIBIAL TRACT
1 Stand with your strong side next to a wall and your weak leg a little distance behind the strong one. Rest most of your weight on your strong leg.
2 Roll on to the outside edge of your weak foot and push the hip on that side out to promote a stretch down the outside of the thigh. Don't push your hips forward and avoid twisting your waist. Hold, relax and repeat.

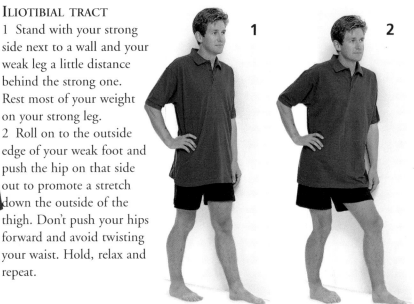

WALL SIT

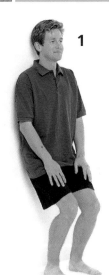

STRENGTHENING QUADRICEPS & HAMSTRINGS
1 Stand with your back against a wall, legs slightly apart, feet parallel and away from the wall. Keeping your bottom and shoulders against the wall, slide down to a "sitting" position with knees bent (aim for a 45-degree angle).
2 Transfer your weight from side to side so that each leg takes the weight alternately.

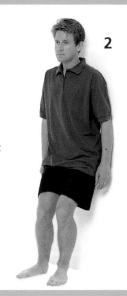

STRAIGHT LEG LIFT

STRENGTHENING QUADRICEPS
Lie on your back with legs straight and toes pointing up. Pull your stomach up and in and use your thigh muscles to lift your leg 45 degrees. Repeat.

HAMSTRING FLICKS

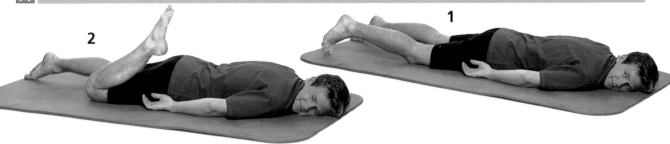

1 Lie on your front with your head to one side and your arms relaxed. Keep the foot of your strong leg flat on the floor and tuck the toes of your weak foot under.
2 Quickly bend your weak knee, flicking your foot up toward your buttock. Relax and repeat.

HAMSTRING SCRUNCH

1 Start in the same position as for the Hamstring Flicks above, this time placing a weight around the ankle of your weak leg.
2 Slowly bend your weak knee, taking your foot up toward your buttock. Relax and repeat.

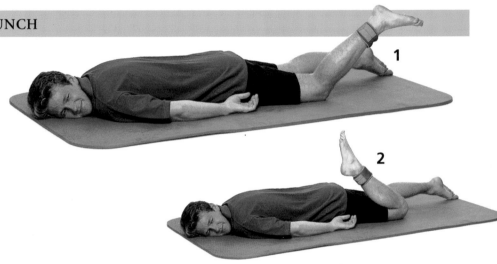

THIGH SCRUNCH

ECCENTRIC QUADRICEPS
1 Pass an elastic exercise band under your weak instep, loop it across the mid-foot in a figure of eight and hold the ends firmly. Lie on your front with your head to one side. Keep your other foot on the floor.
2 Slowly bend your knee, taking your foot up to your buttock; then push against the band to straighten your leg, working the muscle at the front of the thigh. Relax and repeat.

KNEE PUSH

Sit on a chair with your knees at an angle of 90 degrees and your feet resting on the floor. Place the heel of your strong foot into the instep of your weak one and try to move your weak foot by pushing against the strong one. Push from the knee, working the muscle on the inside of the thigh. Hold, relax and repeat.

⚐ THIGH PUSH

Sit on a table, using your hands to support yourself. Push the heel of the foot on your strong side against the instep of your weak one. Tighten your thigh muscles and push your legs against each other. Hold, then relax. Alternate feet and repeat the same exercise, gradually bringing your legs up to the horizontal as you repeat and change the position of your feet.

⚐ DEEP SQUAT

Stand between two chairs, with your feet facing forward. Let your arms bend and your legs squat, lifting your heels off the floor and keeping your feet straight – don't roll on to your instep. This exercise is good for balancing and strengthening the whole leg.

⚐ KNEE BENDS

Stand with knees slightly apart. Pull your stomach up and in and tighten your buttocks. Bend your knees and keep your legs "in line" so that as you look down the kneecap is over the second toe. (Check your position in a mirror.) Keep the arches of your feet up and knees facing forward.

⚐ KNEE LOCK

1 Sit on the floor with your legs out in front of you, hands on the floor for support and a folded towel or two under your weak knee. With your weak foot facing forward and toes pointing up, firmly straighten your knee by tightening the thigh muscles. Feel the muscles working on the front of your thigh.
2 Variation: repeat with your foot facing outward.

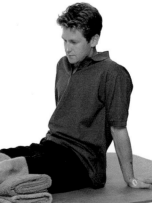

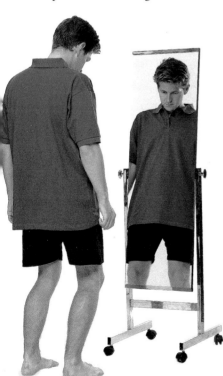

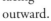

ADVANCED EXERCISES

By the time you progress to these exercises, you should have almost the normal range of movement. Aim for smooth, controlled movements – if you cannot achieve these, continue to do the intermediate exercises for a little longer.

 SQUAT

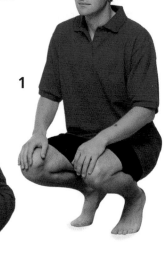

1

1 Squat with your feet slightly apart and facing forward. Lift your heels off the floor. Hold, relax and repeat.
2 Variations: Turn your feet outward and keep your heels flat on the floor; hold, relax and repeat. Turn your feet inward and lift your heels off the floor, hold, relax and repeat.

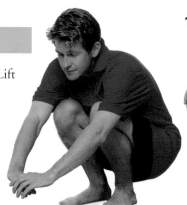

2

 KNEEL TWIST

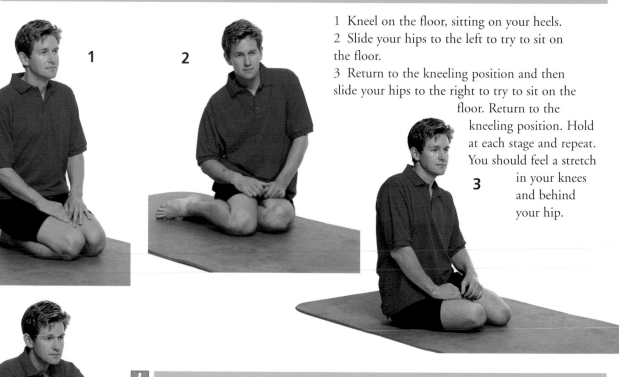

1

2

1 Kneel on the floor, sitting on your heels.
2 Slide your hips to the left to try to sit on the floor.
3 Return to the kneeling position and then slide your hips to the right to try to sit on the floor. Return to the kneeling position. Hold at each stage and repeat. You should feel a stretch in your knees and behind your hip.

3

KNEE STRETCH

Sit on the floor with your legs stretched out in front of you. Put your hands under your knees to compare the gap between the floor and the weak and strong knee. Tighten your thigh to push your weak leg down at the knee and make the gap as similar as possible to the one under the strong knee. Hold for a few seconds.

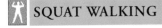 SQUAT WALKING

1 Squat with your feet slightly apart, heels raised off the floor and hands on your knees for balance.
2 Walk 5 to 10 steps in this position. This strengthens the thigh muscles, improves balance and increases mobility in the knee joint.

1

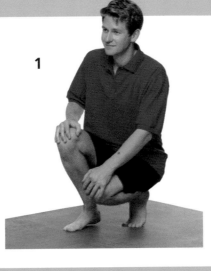

2

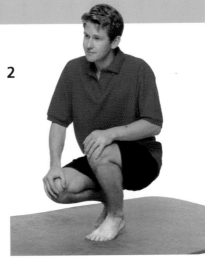

1

STRAIGHT-LEGGED SLUMP

1 Sit up straight with your legs stretched out in front of you and your hands on your knees.
2 Keeping your legs straight, slump through your back and hips to lean forward over your legs. Hold for a few seconds. This increases flexibility through your legs and up into your back.

2

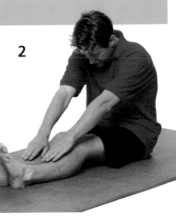

KNEE STRETCH

Lie on your back in a doorway, so that your strong leg is through the doorway and your weak leg is raised and leaning against the wall. Tighten the front of your raised thigh to help relax the muscles at the back of the thigh. Sustain the hold, then relax – allowing the leg to bend – and repeat. Your strong leg should be relaxed and your buttocks on the floor and as close to the wall as possible.

THIGH STRETCH

FEMORAL STRETCH
Stand with your weak knee bent and hold your foot close enough to your buttock for you to feel a stretch in the front of your thigh. Hold your stomach up and in. Relax and repeat.

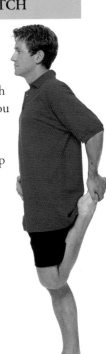

BALANCE

PROPRIOCEPTION

1 Stand on your weak leg with the knee slightly bent so that it leans forward over your foot. Bend your other knee and lift the foot clear of the ground.

2. Keeping your knees apart, twist your torso from the shoulders, using your weak leg to "balance" you. Repeat.

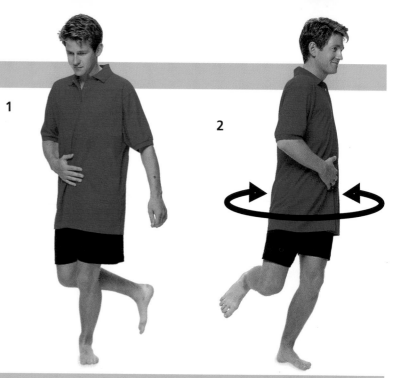

 ## KNEEL UPS

Kneel, sitting on your heels. Raise your body to make a 90-degree angle at the knee. Repeat until fatigued. Variation: Squat with your heels off the floor and raise your body as before.

 ## HAMSTRING FLICKS

With an ankle weight on your weak leg, lie on your front with your head to one side. Keeping your strong foot resting on the floor, quickly bend your weak knee, flicking your foot up toward your buttock. Repeat in short bursts until fatigued.

STEP-UPS, STEP-DOWNS

1 Step up on to a block with your weak foot.

2 Bring your strong foot up on to the block. Step back down with your weak foot and follow with your strong foot. Repeat until fatigued, finding your own pace.

3 & 4 Starting on the block, step down (forward) with your strong foot, follow with your weak foot, then step back up again. Repeat until fatigued.

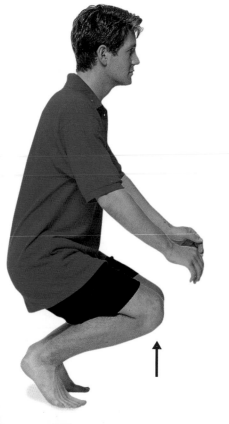

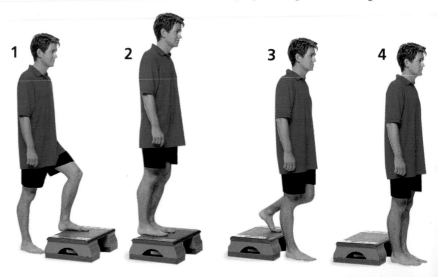

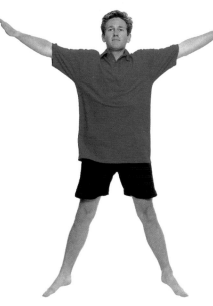

STAR JUMPS

Stand with your body straight but relaxed and your arms hanging at your sides. Jump, quickly opening your arms and legs, and bringing them back in as you land. Repeat until fatigued.

RUNNING

Run on the spot until fatigued, bending your knees gently. This and the other exercises on this page help to build up strength in the knees.

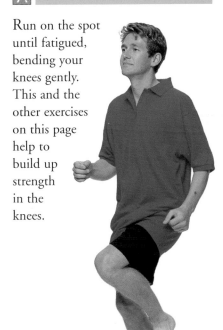

HIGH STEPPING

With your knees bent and coming up as high as you can bring them, run on the spot until fatigued.

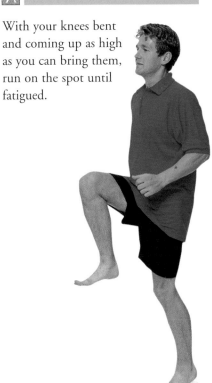

BUNNY HOPS

Hold on to a step or block, squatting on your heels. Keeping hold of the block, jump to one side of it, then to the other. Repeat until fatigued.

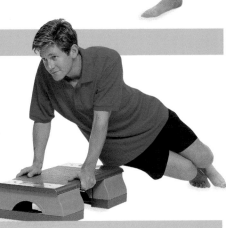

RUNNING STARTS

Start with your hands on the floor, under your shoulders. Keeping one leg stretched out behind you, bend your other leg so that the knee comes up toward your arms. Then quickly reverse the position of the legs. Repeat this movement, finding your own pace, until fatigued.

WALL SKIING

Stand with your back to a wall, with your feet one hip's width apart. Squeeze your buttocks and bend your knees to an angle of 90 degrees, with your back and shoulders against the wall. Try to keep your feet parallel and transfer your weight from side to side to keep your knees moving. Repeat until fatigued. This is particularly useful for strengthening the quadriceps muscles at the front of the thighs.

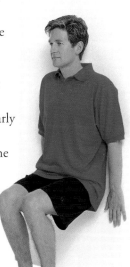

Hip Exercises

The hip is a ball and socket joint, which means that it can move in several directions but remain stable. Western living doesn't put much demand on the hip in terms of mobility, and as the joint is not being put through its full range of movement regularly, the surfaces are not lubricated and the muscles may tighten up and restrict movement. The typical pattern is to lose side swing, back swing and the ability to turn the leg out. If you find these movements difficult, just take your time and emphasize the flexibility exercises. As movement becomes easier, it is important to get the muscles around the hip active. Sometimes these muscles are lazy and your lower back has to compensate. The gluteal muscles (in the buttocks) respond well to exercise and when they are in good working order you can rest assured that your spine is not being put under undue strain.

HOW TO GET STARTED

• Start with the beginners' exercises for mobility. If you find them difficult, concentrate on the beginners' exercises for flexibility, then go back to those for mobility before attempting those for strength and stability. Once they are all easy, move on to the intermediate level.

• If you find an exercise difficult – either because it hurts or because you cannot do the movement – you have identified a problem area. Work through the rest of the exercises at that level and see if any more are difficult. Repeat those particular exercises every day.

• Work on one level of exercises only. Do not attempt any at the intermediate level until you can do all the beginners' exercises comfortably. The same applies when you progress from the intermediate to the advanced level.

MOBILITY

BEGINNER
Hip bend	40
Outward slide	40
Inward slide	40
Inward rotation	40
Hip extension	41
Turn-out rotation	41
Rotations	41
Four-point stretch	41

INTERMEDIATE
Bent knee fall-out	46
Outward slide	46
Hip stretch	46
Outward rotation	46
Knee bend	47
Seated kneel	47
Pelvic thrust	47
Hip quadrant	47

ADVANCED
Sideways stretch	52
Hip stretch	52
Squat	52

FLEXIBILITY

BEGINNER
Prone knee bend	42
Hip stretch	42
Pelvic tilt	42
Sideways knee bend	42
"The waiter's bow"	43
Hip stretches	43

INTERMEDIATE
Seated twist	48
Hip stretch	48
Buttock stretch	48
Prone knee bend	48
Sitting stretch	49
Hip extensions	49
Four-point kneel	49

ADVANCED
Sideways knee bend	52
Seated twist	53
Knee bend	53
Foot roll	53
Sitting slump	53
Four-point kneel	54

STRENGTH & STABILITY

BEGINNER
Trunk stability & hamstring lengthening	43
Heel drag	44
Bent leg extensions	44
Bent leg raises	44
Bent leg lift	44
Pelvic squeeze	45
Knee swing	45
Hip twist	45
Knee bends	45
Weight transference	45

INTERMEDIATE
Kneel twist	50
Straight leg raises	50
Buttock walk	50
Hip adduction	50
Leg raises	51
Knee push	51
Bent knee drops	51

ADVANCED
Two-point kneel	54
Three-point kneel	54
Arms & legs lift	54
Buttock walk	54
Star jumps	55
Scissors	55
Running starts	55
Running	55
Squat thrusts	55
Step-ups	55

BEGINNERS' EXERCISES

These exercises aim to introduce early mobility in all directions at the hip joint, while encouraging muscle control of the movements and flexibility in the soft tissues around the hip. With each exercise, hold and repeat only as long as is comfortable.

HIP BEND

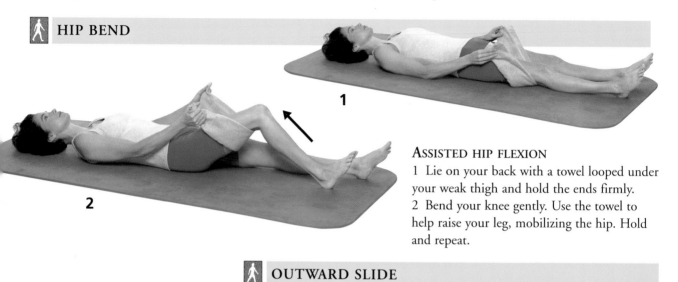

1

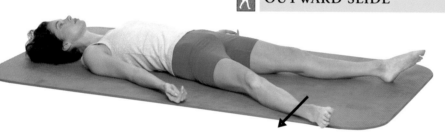

2

ASSISTED HIP FLEXION
1 Lie on your back with a towel looped under your weak thigh and hold the ends firmly.
2 Bend your knee gently. Use the towel to help raise your leg, mobilizing the hip. Hold and repeat.

OUTWARD SLIDE

HIP ABDUCTION
Lie on your back and slide your weak leg outward, keeping it straight but relaxed. Do not rotate your leg at the hip. Repeat.

INWARD SLIDE

NON-WEIGHT BEARING ADDUCTION
1 Lie on your back and cross your strong leg over your weak one, placing the foot flat on the floor close to the weak knee.
2 Keeping your weak leg straight and the heel on the floor, gently move it away from the strong foot. Repeat.

1

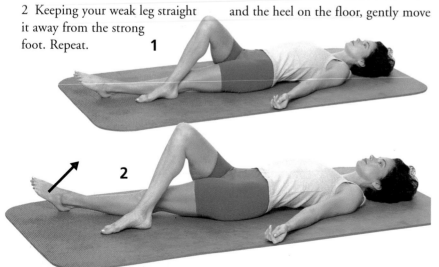

2

INWARD ROTATION

MEDIAL ROTATION
Lie on your back and keep your strong leg straight. Moving from the hip, gently turn the whole of your weak leg inward, taking the inside of your foot as close to the floor as possible. Roll the leg back and repeat.

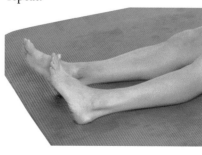

HIP EXTENSION

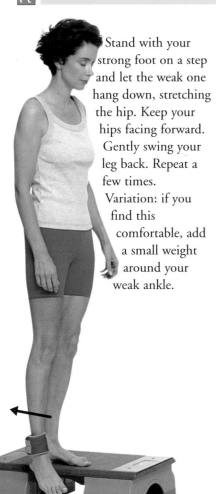

Stand with your strong foot on a step and let the weak one hang down, stretching the hip. Keep your hips facing forward. Gently swing your leg back. Repeat a few times.
Variation: if you find this comfortable, add a small weight around your weak ankle.

TURN-OUT ROTATION

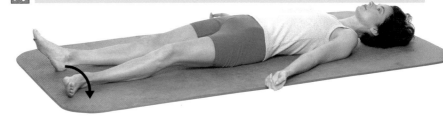

LATERAL ROTATION

Lie on your back. Moving from the hip and keeping your strong leg straight, gently turn the whole of your weak leg out, taking the outside of the foot as close to the floor as possible. Roll your leg back and repeat.

ROTATIONS

MEDIAL AND LATERAL ROTATION WITH KNEE FLEXION

1 Lie on your front with two pillows under your hips and your arms bent on the floor. Bend your weak knee to 90 degrees.
2 Keeping your thigh on the floor, turn your lower leg out, then in. Repeat.

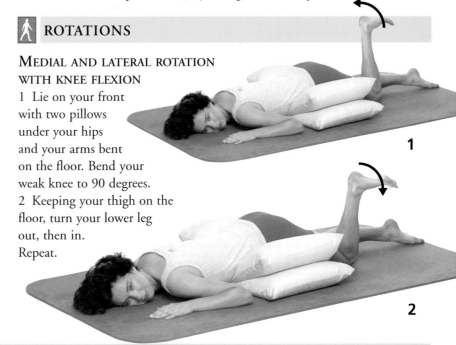

FOUR-POINT STRETCH

PARTIAL WEIGHT-BEARING HIP FLEXION

1 Start on your hands and knees, with your back and arms straight.

2 Gently rock back toward your heels. Hold and repeat.

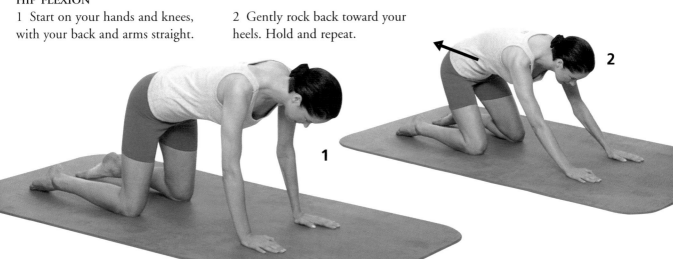

PRONE KNEE BEND

1 Lie on your front with your face to the side and your arms bent on the floor. Place a couple of pillows under your hips.
2 Bend the knee of your weak leg so that the foot comes up toward your buttock, allowing the muscles that

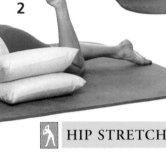

1

run over the front of the hip and into the thigh to lengthen. Hold and repeat.

2

PELVIC TILT

Standing with your back against a wall, tilt your pelvis up and back. Hold and repeat. As you do this you will feel the curve in the small of your back flatten and your stomach muscles pull up and in.

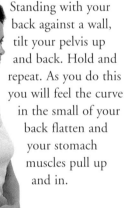

HIP STRETCH

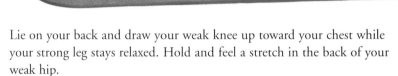

Lie on your back and draw your weak knee up toward your chest while your strong leg stays relaxed. Hold and feel a stretch in the back of your weak hip.

SIDEWAYS KNEE BEND

BENT KNEE FALL-OUT
Sit on the floor with your strong leg straight out in front of you and the foot of your weak side against your calf just below the knee. Put a rolled-up towel under your weak knee to support it. Hold for as long as is comfortable.

   This exercise lengthens muscles on the inside of the thigh and helps hip mobility. When you feel able to – as the soft tissues lengthen – reduce the height of the towel, allowing the knee to drop down further.

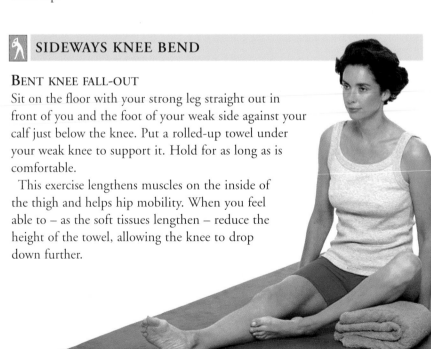

"THE WAITER'S BOW"

HIP & HAMSTRING STRETCH

1 Stand with both hands leaning on a table, legs straight and elbows slightly bent.

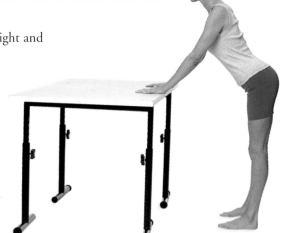

2 Push back gently, so that your hips bend. Don't bend at the waist – stick your bottom out, but don't strain your back. Hold. This exercise lengthens the muscles that run behind the hip and the hamstrings.

HIP STRETCH

Lie on your strong side, with a pillow between your knees. Lift your weak knee up and then relax. Contracting and relaxing the outside muscles of the hip and thigh lengthens the stretch in these areas.

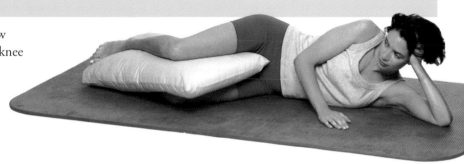

HIP STRETCH

ILIOTIBIAL TRACT

Stand with your strong side against a wall, your strong foot in line with but in front of the weak one, and your strong leg slightly bent, taking most of your weight. Push out through your hips toward your weak side so that you feel a stretch in your outside thigh on that side.

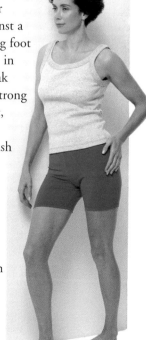

TRUNK STABILITY & HAMSTRING LENGTHENING

Sit on a table, supporting your lower back with your hands. Raise your weak leg 45 degrees, keeping your back steady but not too tense. Repeat. At first you may feel your back "buckle" as you try to stretch your leg. If this happens, relax, correct your back posture and try raising your leg only 20 degrees.

This exercise stabilizes the trunk while stretching the hamstring behind the hip and into the thigh.

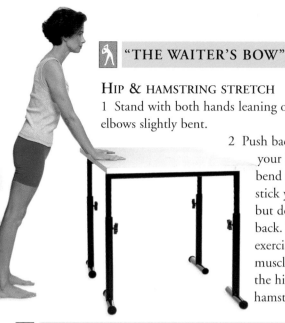

HEEL DRAG

LOWER ABDOMINALS
Lie on your back with abdominal muscles taut (think of pulling your stomach in). Bending your hip and knee to a comfortable position, slowly drag your heel toward your body and push it away again without lifting your foot. Repeat a few times for each leg. This uses the abdominals to keep the trunk stable while the hip and knee move.

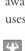 ## BENT LEG EXTENSIONS

HIP EXTENSION & TRUNK STABILITY
Lie on your strong side, supporting yourself on your elbow, with a pillow between your legs. Bend your legs slightly and put your other hand on the floor for balance. With abdominal muscles taut and legs relaxed, slowly move your weak leg behind your body. Hold and repeat. The abdominals keep the trunk stable while the hip extensor muscles move the leg.

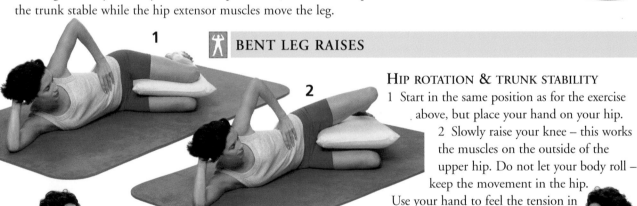

1

2

BENT LEG RAISES

HIP ROTATION & TRUNK STABILITY
1 Start in the same position as for the exercise above, but place your hand on your hip.
2 Slowly raise your knee – this works the muscles on the outside of the upper hip. Do not let your body roll – keep the movement in the hip. Use your hand to feel the tension in your abdominals. Hold for a few seconds and repeat as often as is comfortable.

1

2

BENT LEG LIFT

HIP FLEXION & TRUNK STABILITY
1 Sit on a table and press your hands flat on the table to keep your back straight. Dangle your legs, bending hips and knees at an angle of 90 degrees.
2 Tighten your abdominals and gently lift your weak leg. Hold and repeat. This exercise uses the abdominal muscles to keep the trunk stable while the hip moves.

PELVIC SQUEEZE

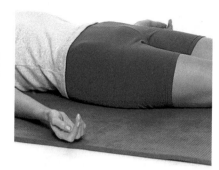

Lie on your back and tighten your abdominals and buttocks, keeping your legs flat on the ground. Variation: sit on a table or high stool and squeeze your buttocks together. Hold for 3 to 5 seconds. Repeat up to 20 times.

KNEE SWING

HIP ROTATION

Sit on a table or high stool. Keeping your legs relaxed, turn the weak leg out (1) and in (2) from the hip. Repeat. This exercise increases hip mobility and strength while stabilizing the trunk.

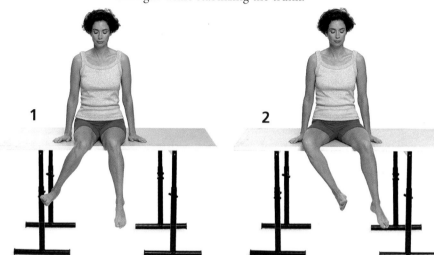

HIP TWIST

Lie on your front and tighten your buttocks. Bend the knee on your weak side to an angle of 90 degrees and let the foot roll out away from your body (1) and back in to the mid-line (2). Repeat. This exercise promotes stability of the trunk and strength in the rotator muscles of the hip.

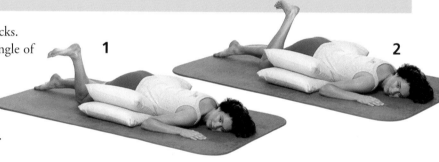

KNEE BENDS

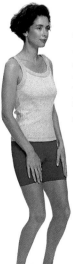

Stand with your back straight and feet and knees facing forward. Gently bend both knees and hold. Straighten your knees and repeat. This exercise coordinates the hip and leg muscles as they control your body weight against the pull of gravity.

WEIGHT TRANSFERENCE

1 Sit on the edge of a chair, with your weak foot flat on the ground, facing forward. Raise your other foot up on to the toes.
2 Keeping your back straight, push down through your strong foot to lift your body up out of the chair, transferring your weight forward on to your weak foot as you stand up. Reverse the movement to sit down. Repeat.

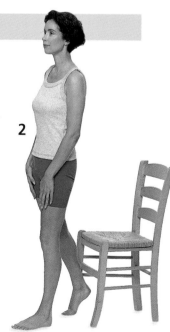

INTERMEDIATE EXERCISES

Do not move on to these exercises until you can do all the beginners' ones easily. Work steadily; don't push yourself to do exercises for which your body is not ready. You should be able to hold positions for longer than a few seconds, and repeat 6 to 8 times.

BENT KNEE FALL-OUT

HIP ABDUCTION, FLEXION & LATERAL ROTATION

Sit on a chair with your weak leg bent and the foot tucked against the opposite thigh. Hold for 10–20 seconds, then repeat. This exercise lengthens muscles on the inside of the thigh and helps hip mobility.

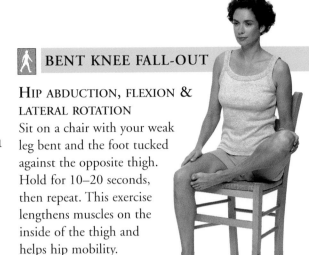

OUTWARD SLIDE

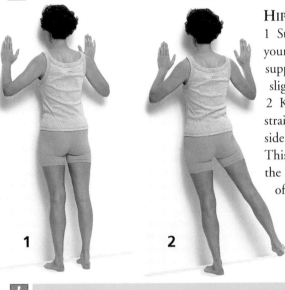

HIP ABDUCTION

1 Stand facing a wall, with your hands on the wall to support you and your feet slightly apart.
2 Keeping your weak leg straight, slide it out to the side and back again. Repeat. This exercise strengthens the muscles on the outside of the hip.

1   **2**

HIP STRETCH

GLUTEUS MAXIMUS

Standing with your strong side next to a wall and your hand on the wall for support, extend your weak leg out behind you. Don't let your back arch. Rest your other hand on your stomach. Keep your abdominals taut so that your trunk is stable and the movement comes from the hip rather than the spine. Hold and repeat.

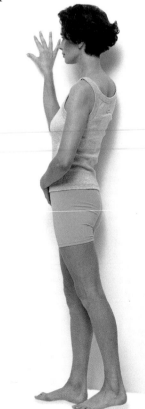

OUTWARD ROTATION

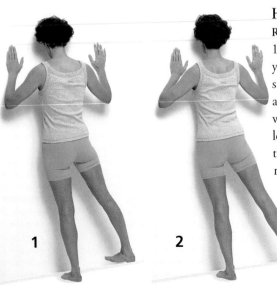

HIP ABDUCTION/ ROTATION

1 Stand facing a wall, with your hands on the wall to support you and feet slightly apart. Turn the foot on your weak side in, then lift that leg out to the side. Return to the starting position and repeat. This coordinates and strengthens the muscles on the outside of the hip.
2 Variation: turn your foot out, then lift your leg out to the side.

1   **2**

KNEE BEND

PARTIAL WEIGHT-BEARING HIP FLEXION

1 Stand facing a chair. Step up on to the chair with your weak foot, keeping the other foot on the floor.
2 Holding on to the chair, bend the supporting leg and lean gently forward on to your weak leg so that your hip and knee bend further and the knee comes up toward your chest. Feel the movement at the front of your hip. Sustain the position for up to 10 seconds.

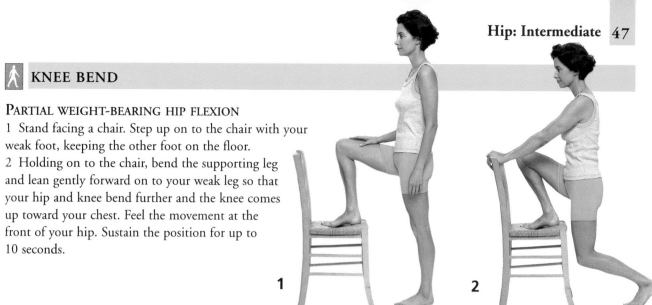

SEATED KNEEL

WEIGHT TRANSFERENCE

1 Kneel down, sitting on your heels.
2 Shift your hips over to the left side and hold. Try to take your bottom to the floor.
3 Then shift your hips to the right side and hold. Repeat the sequence. This exercise coordinates hip and trunk muscle work while improving hip mobility.

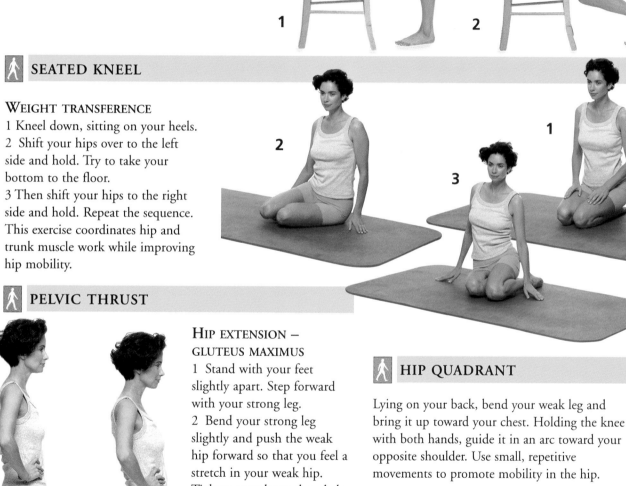

PELVIC THRUST

HIP EXTENSION –
GLUTEUS MAXIMUS

1 Stand with your feet slightly apart. Step forward with your strong leg.
2 Bend your strong leg slightly and push the weak hip forward so that you feel a stretch in your weak hip. Tighten your buttock to help the movement.

HIP QUADRANT

Lying on your back, bend your weak leg and bring it up toward your chest. Holding the knee with both hands, guide it in an arc toward your opposite shoulder. Use small, repetitive movements to promote mobility in the hip.

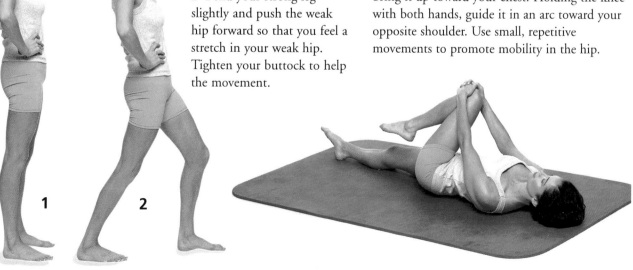

SEATED TWIST

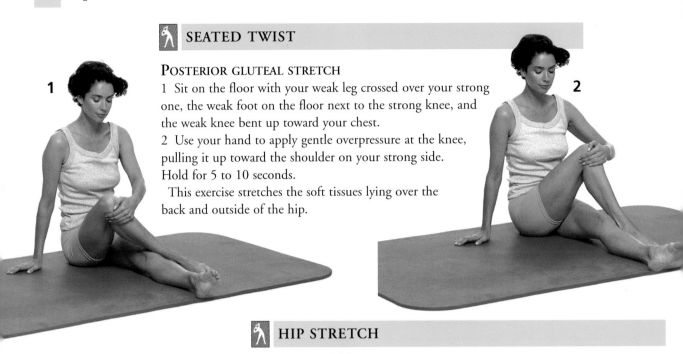

POSTERIOR GLUTEAL STRETCH

1 Sit on the floor with your weak leg crossed over your strong one, the weak foot on the floor next to the strong knee, and the weak knee bent up toward your chest.

2 Use your hand to apply gentle overpressure at the knee, pulling it up toward the shoulder on your strong side. Hold for 5 to 10 seconds.

This exercise stretches the soft tissues lying over the back and outside of the hip.

HIP STRETCH

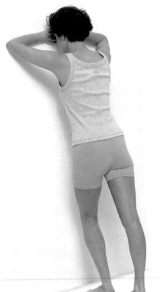

1 Face a wall with your weak leg straight and behind the strong one, which is slightly bent. Push against the wall with your forearms. Hold, feeling a stretch in the outside thigh.

2 Variation: cross your weak foot over behind your strong one.

BUTTOCK STRETCH

POSTERIOR HIP STRETCH

Lie with your strong leg vertically against a wall, with your bottom as close to the wall as possible. Bend your weak knee and place your ankle on the opposite thigh, just above the knee. Bend your strong knee slightly and hold. This is a strong stretch that will be felt on the outside of the weak hip.

PRONE KNEE BEND

Lie on your front with your legs straight and toes gently pointed. Bend your weak knee so that the foot comes up toward the buttock, to allow the muscles that run over the front of the hip and into the thigh to lengthen. Hold, relax and repeat.

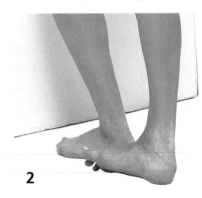

SITTING STRETCH

LATERAL STRETCH

1 Sit with your legs stretched out in front of you, keeping your back straight.
2 Turn your weak leg in and pull the toes up toward your body. Hold and feel a stretch along the outside of your leg.

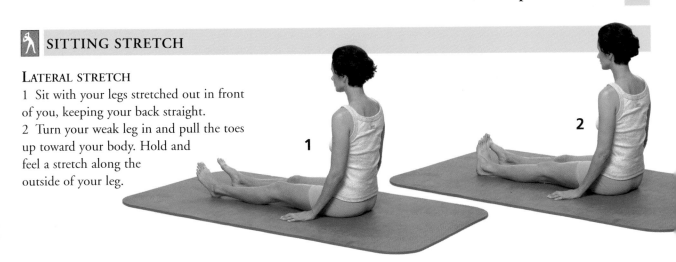

HIP EXTENSIONS

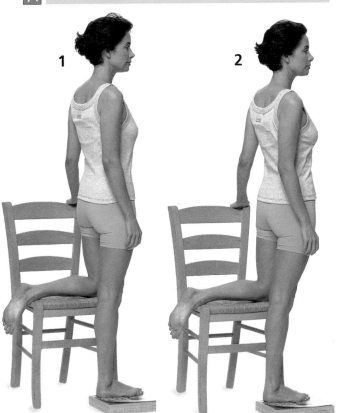

ANTERIOR HIP STRETCH

1 Stand in front of a chair and place your weak knee on the seat with your foot over the edge. If the chair is not quite the right height, stand on a telephone book or other solid object so that your hips are level.
2 Lean forward from the hip and feel a stretch at the front of your hip and thigh. Hold for 5 to 10 seconds. This exercise promotes further lengthening of the soft tissues in front of the hip and into the front of the thigh.

FOUR-POINT KNEEL

POSTERO-LATERAL GLUTEAL STRETCH

Start on your hands and knees, with your arms taking a lot of your weight (1). Without moving your hands, sit back toward your heels. Move your buttocks first toward the left side (2), then toward the right (3). Repeat. This promotes a further stretch of the soft tissues behind the hip joint.

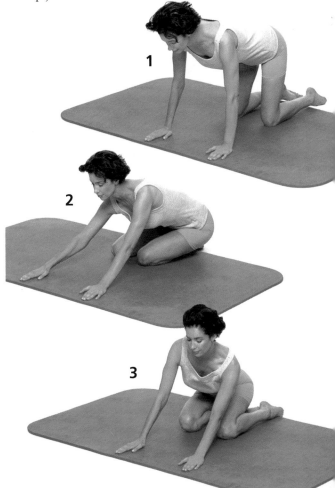

KNEEL TWIST

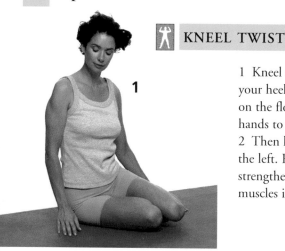

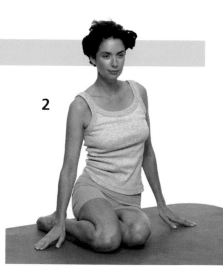

1 Kneel on the floor, sitting back on your heels. Lift your buttocks and sit on the floor to the right. Use your hands to balance you if necessary.
2 Then lift your buttocks and sit to the left. Repeat. This exercise strengthens and coordinates the muscles in the hip and thigh.

STRAIGHT LEG RAISES

HIP FLEXION CONTROL

1 Lie on your back with your feet relaxed.
2 Lift your weak leg to an angle of about 45 degrees, then slowly bring it down again. Repeat. Place your fingers on the top of your femur (thigh bone) to check the axis of movement in the hip.

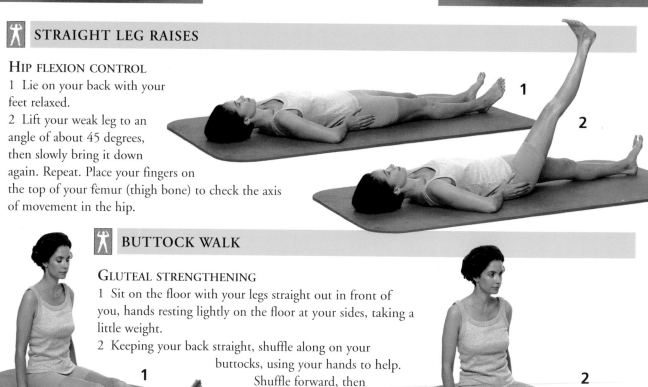

BUTTOCK WALK

GLUTEAL STRENGTHENING

1 Sit on the floor with your legs straight out in front of you, hands resting lightly on the floor at your sides, taking a little weight.
2 Keeping your back straight, shuffle along on your buttocks, using your hands to help. Shuffle forward, then backward.

HIP ADDUCTION

Lie on your weak side, supporting your head on your hand and with the other hand on the floor for balance. Bend your strong leg and rest it on the floor in front of your weak one. Keeping your weak leg straight, lift it up from the floor to strengthen the muscles of the inner thigh.

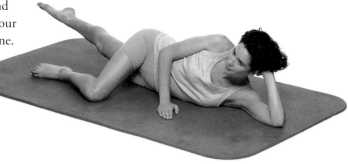

LEG RAISES

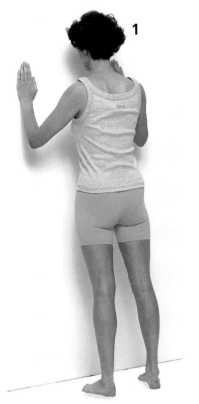

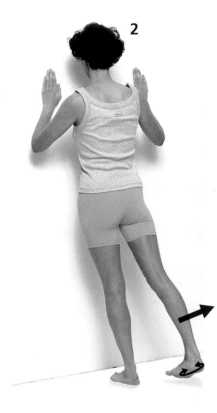

HIP ABDUCTORS

Stand facing a wall, with hands resting lightly on it, elbows bent, weak leg slightly out to the side and foot turned in (1). Lift your leg out sideways, keeping your abdominals taut so that the movement comes from the hip (2). Repeat. You should feel the muscles working on the outside of your hip.

KNEE PUSH

HIP ABDUCTORS

Stand with your weak side leaning against a wall, with the leg slightly bent, foot off the floor and knee and lower leg resting against the wall. Push your knee into the wall and tense your other leg to resist the turning force this creates. Repeat the exercise with your other side next to the wall. Be careful not to tilt your body away from the wall.

 ## BENT KNEE DROPS

Lie on your front, with your abdominal muscles and buttocks taut and a small weight around your weak ankle. Bend your weak knee to an angle of 90 degrees. Keeping your thigh resting on the floor, roll your bent leg slowly out to the side (1) and back again (2). Repeat. This exercise coordinates trunk stability with hip movement, strengthening the hip rotator muscles.

ADVANCED EXERCISES

These exercises promote increasing mobility, flexibility and strength as the joints and soft tissues heal. You should be able to achieve something close to a full range of movement in the hip. Repeat the strengthening exercises until fatigued.

 SIDEWAYS KNEE BEND

BENT KNEE FALL-OUT WITH OVERPRESSURE
Sit on the floor with your strong leg straight out in front of you and your weak leg bent so that the foot is flat against the inside of the opposite leg, as high up as it will go comfortably. Push down gently on your weak knee with your hand to increase the movement. Hold, relax and repeat. Feel a stretch in your inner thigh and groin.

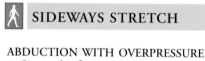 **SIDEWAYS STRETCH**

ABDUCTION WITH OVERPRESSURE
1 Sit on the floor with legs out in front of you.
2 Slide your weak leg to the side, using your hand to stretch it as far as possible. Hold, relax and repeat. Feel a stretch in your inner thigh and groin.

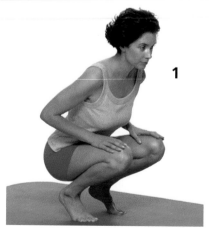

 HIP STRETCH

EXTENSION
Stand beside a chair, with your weak knee on the seat and your foot over the edge. If the chair is not quite at the right height, stand on a telephone book or similar solid object so that your hips are level. Tighten your buttocks and lean forward from the hip, using your hands to increase the movement by pushing through your lower back and hip, so that you feel the stretch at the front of your hip and thigh.

 SQUAT

1 Squat on the floor with your heels raised. Keep your hands off the ground. Hold for as long as you can.
2 Variation: keep your heels on the ground. Use your arms to help maintain the position. Hold. Feel a stretch in the back of your hips.

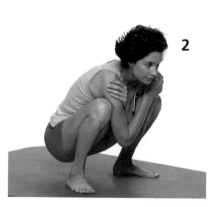

SEATED TWIST

POSTERIOR GLUTEAL STRETCH

Sit on the floor with your weak leg crossed over your strong one, the weak foot flat on the floor next to the strong knee, and the weak knee bent up toward your chest. Use your strong hand to apply overpressure at the knee, pulling it in toward the shoulder on your strong side. Hold for 5 to 10 seconds.

This promotes a greater degree of stretch in the soft tissues lying over the back and outside of the hip.

KNEE BEND

PRONE KNEE BEND WITH OVERPRESSURE

Lying on your front on the floor, bend your weak knee and take hold of the foot, drawing it toward your buttock. Hold, relax and repeat.

FOOT ROLL

ADDUCTOR STRETCH

Stand with your feet apart, your strong leg bent and your weak leg straight. Roll your weight on to the inside edge of your weak foot. Bend your strong knee to increase the stretch on the inside of your weak thigh.

SITTING SLUMP

1 Sit on the floor with your legs straight out in front of you.
2 Keeping your chin tucked in, slump your torso forward and reach toward your toes with your hands. This increases flexibility throughout the spine and down into the legs.

1

2

FOUR-POINT KNEEL

1

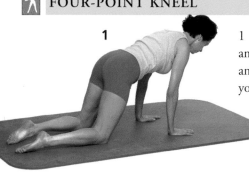

1 Kneel on all fours with your knees at an angle of 90 degrees and your back and arms straight. Lean forward, so that your weight is over your hands. Hold.

2 Lean backward. Hold. This improves balance and coordinates hip stability muscles.

2

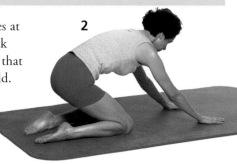

TWO-POINT KNEEL

HIP STABILITY

Balance on your weak knee and opposite hand, with the opposite arm and leg outstretched. Balance in this position. Then reverse the position, balancing on your strong knee and opposite hand. Hold.
This exercise coordinates and strengthens the stabilizing muscles in the hip

THREE-POINT KNEEL

HIP ABDUCTION

Kneel on all fours with your knees at an angle of 90 degrees and your back straight. Lift your weak leg up to the side – aim to get the leg level with the hip. Hold. Swap legs and repeat. When kneeling on your weak leg, make sure that you stay steady and do not drift over to the side.

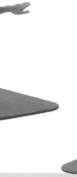

ARMS & LEGS LIFT

Lie face down with your arms stretched by your side and your head on the floor. Lift your arms and legs, holding them off the ground for a count of 10. Relax and repeat.
This exercise works your back muscles and the muscles in the back of your legs.

BUTTOCK WALK

GLUTEAL STRENGTH

Sit on the floor with your legs straight out in front of you and your arms folded. Shuffle forward across the floor, then back. Repeat until fatigued. This strengthens the muscles in your buttocks.

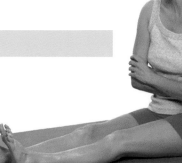

⚹ STAR JUMPS

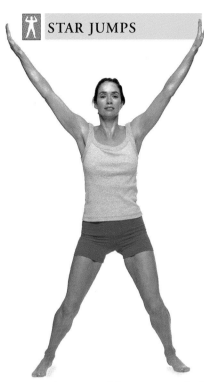

Jump with arms and legs outstretched. Land gently, letting your hips and knees bend. Repeat until fatigued.

⚹ SCISSORS

HIP FLEXION & ADDUCTION
Sit on the floor with legs out in front of you. Leaning back on your elbows, lift your legs up as high as possible. Cross back and forth in a scissors motion, moving them up and down without touching the ground. Keep stomach pulled up and in. Repeat as often as you can.

⚹ RUNNING STARTS

Start with your hands on the floor under your shoulders. Keeping one leg stretched out behind you, jump so that the other leg comes up between your arms with the toes tucked under, not stretched out behind. Jump repeatedly, alternating legs, until fatigued. This strengthens the muscles in the hips and legs.

⚹ RUNNING

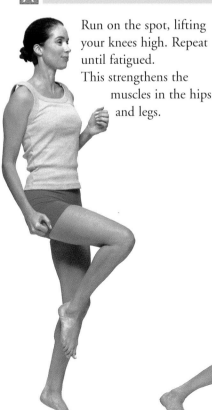

Run on the spot, lifting your knees high. Repeat until fatigued. This strengthens the muscles in the hips and legs.

⚹ SQUAT THRUSTS

1

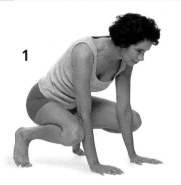

2

1 Start in a wide squat, with your knees outside your elbows.
2 Jump back, thrusting your legs apart, then return to the starting position. Keep your back straight. Repeat.

⚹ STEP-UPS

Step up on to a step or block, leading with your weak leg. Then step down again, also leading with your weak leg. After a few steps, switch legs so that you lead up and down with your strong leg. Repeat until fatigued.

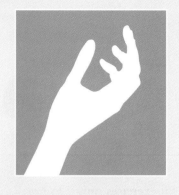

Wrist & Hand Exercises

Injuries to the wrist and hand commonly occur following a fall. Reaching out instinctively to break the fall often damages the wrist, resulting either in a fracture or in a strain to the ligaments that hold the bones together. Initially, there will be swelling and bruising; then, as the tissues heal, movement will feel restricted and painful. If the wrist has been in plaster, the hand and wrist often feel vulnerable when the plaster comes off; any movement may be difficult and painful.

For these injuries it is important to start with simple movements and progress gently. Be prepared for some soreness, but expect this to settle a few minutes after you stop exercising.

Arthritis can make the finger joints painful and swollen. At first they are likely to be too sore to exercise, but once the heat and swelling has subsided, gentle exercises help to restore mobility. Consult a professional for advice before you start.

HOW TO GET STARTED

• Start with the beginners' exercises for mobility. If you can do them all easily, try the beginners' exercises for flexibility, then those for strength and stability. If they are all easy, move on to the intermediate level.

• If at any stage you find an exercise is difficult – either because it hurts or because you cannot do the movement – you have identified a problem area. Work through the rest of the exercises at that level and see if any more are difficult. Repeat those particular exercises every day and you should find it becomes easier.

• Work on one level of exercises only. Do not attempt any at the intermediate level until you can do all the beginners' exercises comfortably. The same applies when you progress from the intermediate to the advanced level.

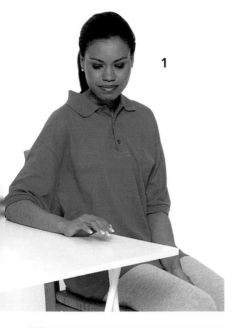

BEGINNERS' EXERCISES

Treat these exercises gently – do not do anything to the point of pain, and hold any position only as long as it is comfortable. You are taking the first steps toward restoring strength and mobility to your wrist and hand.

FOUR-WAY MOVEMENT

EXTENSION, ULNAR & RADIAL DEVIATION
Sit with your elbow bent and your hand and forearm resting on a table, palm down.
1 Moving from the wrist only, lift your hand off the table, then lower it. Repeat.
2 Lift your hand slightly off the table and move from side to side. Do not move your forearm.

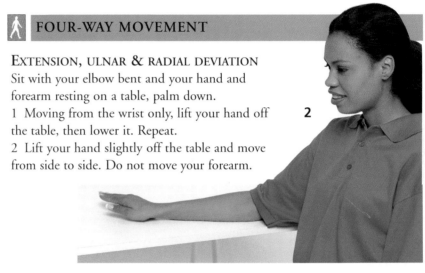

WRIST TWIST

SUPINATION
1 Start in the same position as above. Twist your forearm so that your palm faces upward and curl your fingers in toward your palm.
2 Straighten your fingers and repeat as often as you can without it becoming painful.

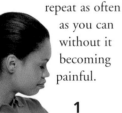

WRIST LIFT

FLEXION
Start in the same position as above but with your palm facing upward, lift your hand off the table. Move from the wrist only – do not lift your arm. Lower and repeat. The three exercises on this page all work to improve mobility in the wrist and forearm.

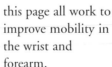

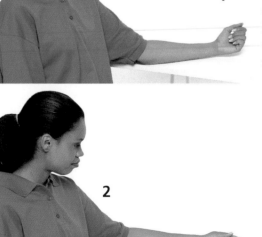

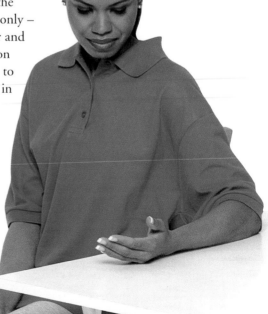

FINGER CURL

FINGER FLEXION & EXTENSION

1 Sit with your elbow bent and your forearm resting on a table, palm up. Curl your fingers in toward your palm – you may not be able to make a tight fist at this stage.

2 Then straighten your fingers as far as they will go. Relax and repeat the sequence.

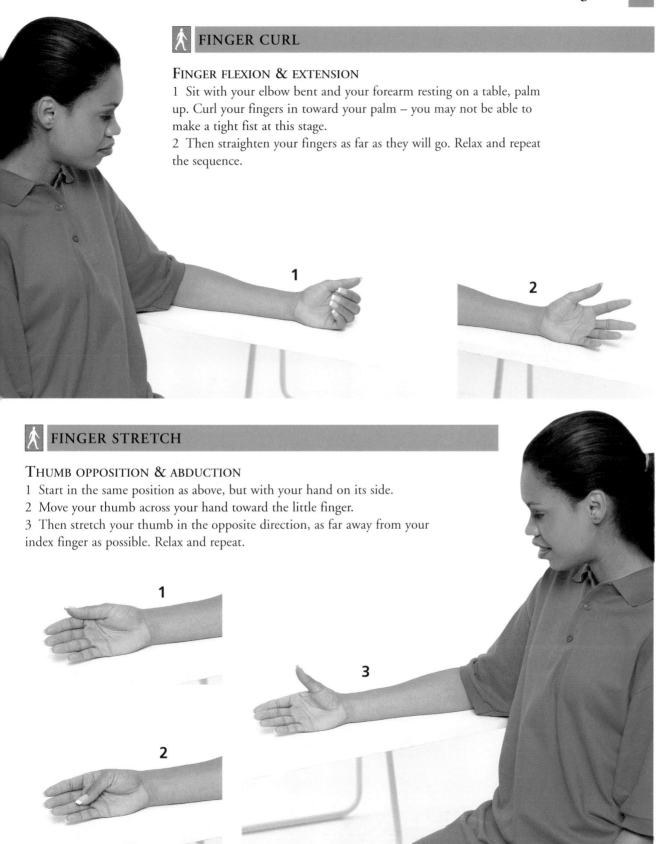

FINGER STRETCH

THUMB OPPOSITION & ABDUCTION

1 Start in the same position as above, but with your hand on its side.

2 Move your thumb across your hand toward the little finger.

3 Then stretch your thumb in the opposite direction, as far away from your index finger as possible. Relax and repeat.

WRIST TWIST

PRONATION & SUPINATION

Stand with your elbow bent and your hand in a loose fist at your mid-line (1). Twist your wrist and forearm so that your hand faces in (2), then out (3).

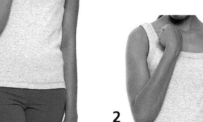

1

2

3

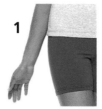 FOUR-WAY WRIST STRETCH

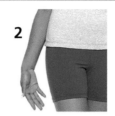

1

2

3

WRIST EXTENSION, FLEXION, ULNAR & RADIAL DEVIATION

With your arm by your side, elbow straight and palm facing forward (1), move from the wrist to bring your hand back, then forward (2). Repeat. With your palm facing down, move your hand diagonally to the right, then to the left (3). Repeat.

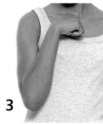

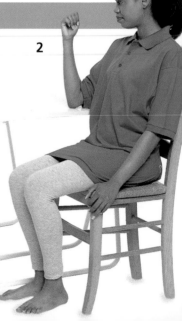

KNUCKLE MASSAGE

SOFT TISSUE MASSAGE

Sitting at a table with your weak arm resting on it, use the fingers of your other hand to massage the area round an affected knuckle. After an injury the tissues sometimes become "bound down". The aim of this exercise is to loosen the tissues over the muscles so that they slide easily over one another.

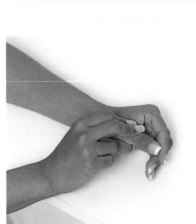

FOREARM STRETCH

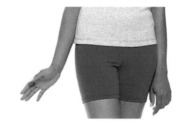

FINGER EXTENSION & ABDUCTION

Stand with your arm by your side and your elbow straight. Bend your fingers back and stretch them as far apart as possible. Relax and repeat.

FINGER CURL & STRETCH

1

FINGER FLEXION & EXTENSION

1 Rest your elbow on a table, keeping your forearm vertical.
2 Curl your fingers in as far as you can without strain, then straighten them.

2

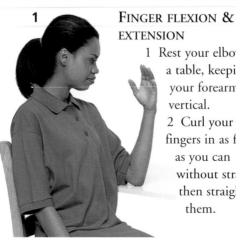

GRIP

RESISTED FINGER FLEXION

Sit at a table with your arm resting
on it, elbow bent. Grip, squeeze and
manipulate a soft ball, lump of play
dough, handful of cotton wool or
the like, making your fingers do
the work.

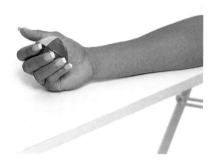

WRIST LIFT

RADIAL DEVIATION

1 Starting in the same position as for the Grip exercise,
left, put your hand on its side with the thumb pointing
upward.
2 Moving from the wrist only, lift your hand off the
table. Relax and repeat.

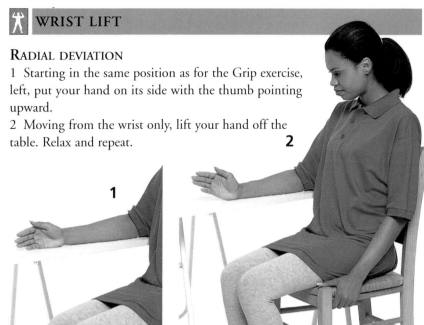

FIVE-FINGER EXERCISE

WRIST EXTENSION, FINGER EXTENSION & CO-ORDINATING FINGER MOVEMENTS

1 Starting in the same position as above, place your palm flat on the table.
2 Moving from the wrist, lift your fingers off the table. Relax and repeat. Then, keeping your palm on the table,
lift and lower one finger at a time. Relax and repeat.
3 Drum your fingers on the table, lifting each finger in turn. Repeat.

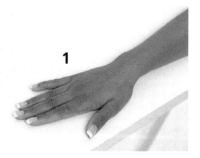
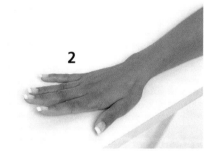
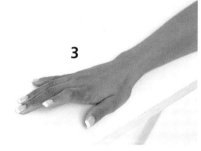

FINGER DEXTERITY

COORDINATING FINGER MOVEMENTS

Starting in the same position as above, touch the tip of your little finger
with your thumb. Move your thumb to the tip of your fourth finger,
then your middle finger and finally your index finger.
Work back the other way and repeat.

INTERMEDIATE EXERCISES

These exercises will promote further strength and mobility in wrist and hand. Do not attempt them until you can do the beginners' ones comfortably. Aim to hold positions for slightly longer than before, and repeat most exercises 6 to 8 times.

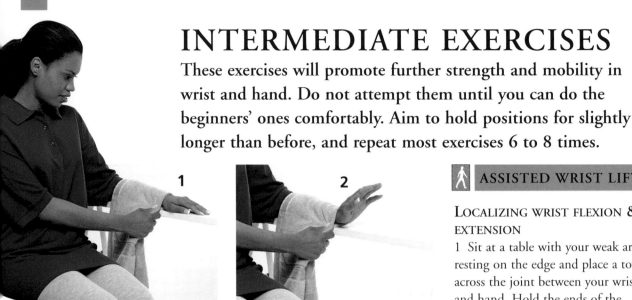

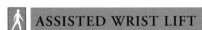

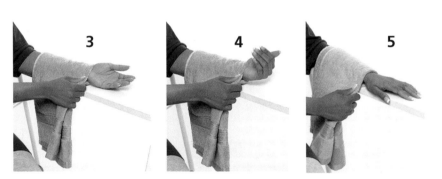

ASSISTED WRIST LIFT

LOCALIZING WRIST FLEXION & EXTENSION

1 Sit at a table with your weak arm resting on the edge and place a towel across the joint between your wrist and hand. Hold the ends of the towel firmly in your other hand.
2 Moving from the wrist only, raise and lower your hand, pushing against the towel.
3 Turn your palm upward.
4 Lift your hand from the wrist, feeling the pressure of the towel.
5 Move the towel up your arm slightly, to the point where the two bones of the forearm (the radius and the ulna) meet the bones of the wrist, and repeat both exercises.

ASSISTED WRIST TWIST

RADIAL & ULNAR DEVIATION, PRONATION & SUPINATION WITH OVERPRESSURE

1 Sit facing a table with the palm of your weak arm facing down. Place the thumb and fingers of your strong hand across the weak wrist.
2 Use the strength in your strong hand to assist in sliding your weak hand from side to side.
3 Still using your strong hand to assist the movement, twist your wrist so that the palm comes slightly upward.
4 Twist your wrist back so that your palm is facing downward. Repeat as often as is comfortable.

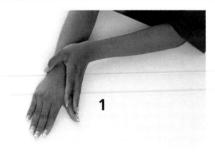

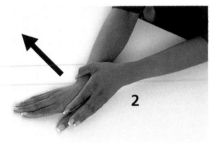

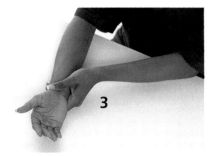

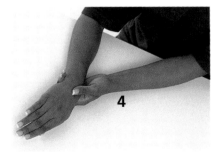

FORWARD LEAN

PARTIAL WEIGHT-BEARING IN EXTENSION

Stand with your feet slightly apart, knees straight and hands flat on a table. With elbows slightly bent, lean forward with your weight on your wrists so that they bend back slightly.

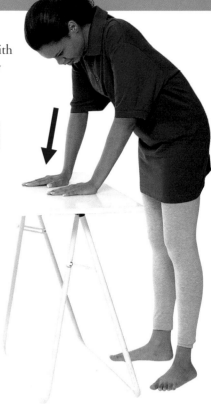

MOBILIZING THUMB, FINGERS & WRIST

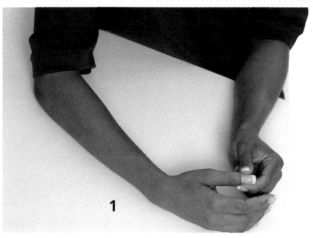

1

FINGER & THUMB FLEXION

1 Sit at a table with your elbow and forearm resting on it, and your weak hand on its side. Use your other hand to massage your thumb and fingers, twisting the thumb toward the rest of the hand, then away from it.

2 With your weak palm facing upward, use your other hand to bend the thumb and all the fingers toward the palm.

3 Repeat, bending each finger individually.

4 With your fingers and thumb curled in toward your palm, cradle your weak hand in your stronger one and use its strength to bend your wrist up as far as it will go without straining. Relax and repeat.

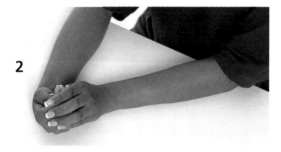

2

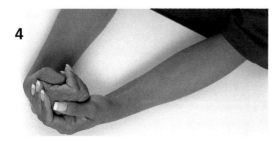

4

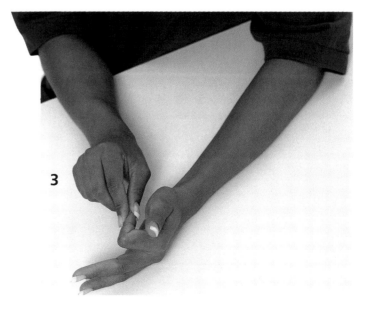

3

WRIST TWIST

PRONATION & SUPINATION

1 Stand with your elbow bent so that your hand is close to your shoulder and faces downward. Curl your fingers to make a loose fist. Moving from the wrist only, twist your hand from side to side. Still moving from the wrist only, lift your hand, then lower it again. Twist your wrist and forearm so that your hand turns in toward your body.
2 Straighten your fingers and bend your hand back from the wrist, stretching your fingers as far apart as they will go, then bend the hand forward again. Repeat the sequence a few times.

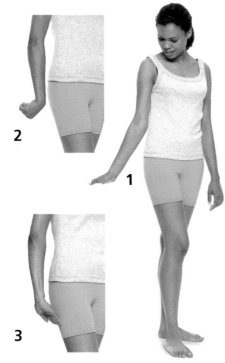

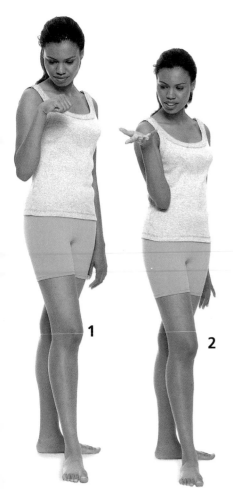

FINGER STRETCH

FINGER MOBILITY; WRIST FLEXION & EXTENSION

1 Stand with your arm hanging loosely by your side. Keeping your elbow as straight as possible, stretch your arm out behind you and slightly to the side – there should be an angle of about 20 to 45 degrees between your arm and your body. Stretch your hand and fingers as far back as they will go.
2 Keeping your hand stretched back, flex your fingers and curl them in toward your palm.
3 Twist your wrist so that your hand is facing in toward your thigh. Relax and repeat.

WRIST SCRUNCHES

RESISTED WRIST & FOREARM MOVEMENTS

Sitting at a table with your arm resting on it and your hand hanging over the edge, wrap an elastic exercise band round your hand, passing it between thumb and index finger. Hold the ends of the band in your other hand, and keep this in the same place throughout so that your weak hand pulls against the pressure of the band.
1 With your palm facing downward, raise your hand from the wrist, then lower.
2 Turn your hand over and repeat the exercise, moving from the wrist to raise and lower the hand a few times.
3 With your hand on its side, point your fingers toward the floor, then raise them as far as they will go and lower them again.
4 Clench your fingers and twist your hand backward and forward, turning your wrist as you do so.

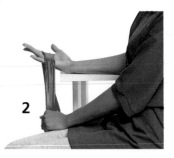

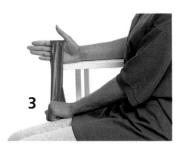

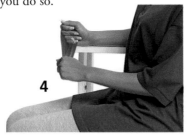

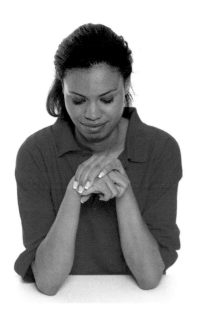

ADVANCED EXERCISES

Progress to these exercises when you can do the intermediate ones comfortably. You should be able to achieve almost the normal range of movement. Repeat the exercises until fatigued.

 WRIST BEND

WRIST FLEXION

Sit at a table with your elbows resting on it and your forearms raised. With your palms facing downward, place the fingers of your strong hand across the back of your weak one. Use your strong hand to press the weak hand gently downward, bending the wrist. Hold this position, then nudge down a little further and hold again.

SIDE-TO-SIDE WRIST BEND

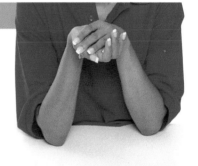

ULNAR & RADIAL DEVIATION

Starting in the same position, turn your palm upward. Place the thumb of your strong hand under your weak hand and the fingers over it. Using your strong hand to help, move your wrist from side to side as far as it will go.

 WRIST TWIST

PRONATION & SUPINATION

Sit with elbows bent and forearms resting on a table. Clasp your wrist with your strong hand and use it to help twist the wrist back and forth so that the palm faces up (1) and then down (2).

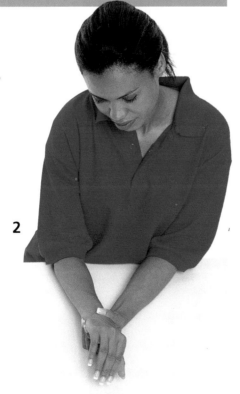

2

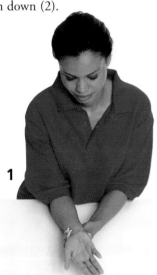

1

HAND STRETCH

FINGER EXTENSION/THUMB OPPOSITION

In the same position as above, with palm up, use your strong hand to push your fingers down as far as they will go comfortably. Then use your strong hand to draw the weak thumb across the palm toward the little finger. Hold, relax and repeat.

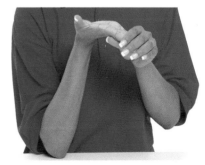

BACKWARD STRETCH

ANTERIOR FLEXIBILITY

1 Stand with your weak arm hanging loosely at your side.

2 Stretch it out behind you and slightly to the side. With your palm facing downward, bend your wrist back and stretch your fingers and thumb back and apart, pulling the back of the hand up. You should feel this exercise stretching the whole arm.

ASSISTED STRETCH

PASSIVE FINGER & WRIST FLEXION

1 Stand with your hands clasped loosely in front of you, the strong hand cupping the weak one.

2 Use your strong hand to bend the fingers of the weak hand in toward the palm. Your weak hand should be passive, yielding to the pressure of the strong one.

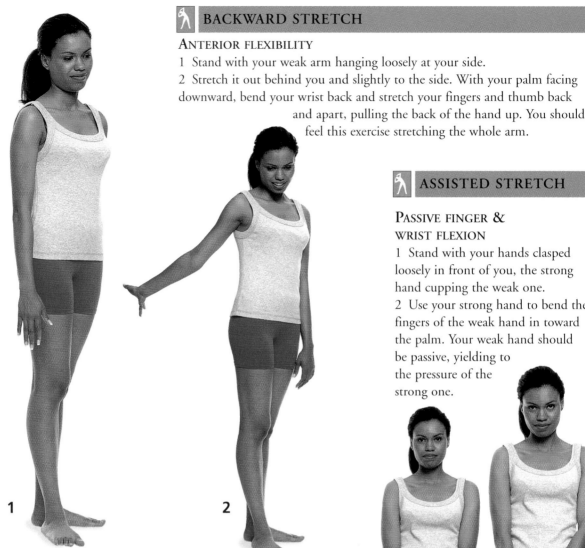

1

2

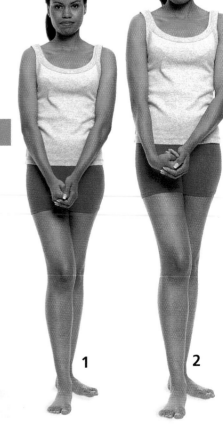

1

2

PRAYING STRETCH

ACTIVE WRIST EXTENSION

Sit at a table with your forearms flat on it and your hands together in a praying position. Keeping your fingers together, pull your forearms away so that you feel a stretch in the front of your wrist.

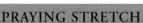

FIVE-FINGER STRETCH

FINGER & THUMB ABDUCTION
Sit with your elbows on a table and your fingertips together. Stretch your fingers as far apart as they will go and feel the stretch in the webbing between each finger.

FINGER & THUMB STRETCH

PASSIVE THUMB ABDUCTION
Starting in the same position as above, place the tips of your index fingers and thumbs together to form a "steeple". Stretch your index fingers and thumbs as far apart as they will go and feel the stretch in the webbing between them.

INDIVIDUAL FINGER STRETCH

PASSIVE ABDUCTION STRETCH
Starting in the same position as above, use your strong hand to spread the index finger and third finger of your weak hand as far apart as they will go. Repeat with the third and fourth fingers, then the fourth and little fingers.

RESISTED TWIST

GRIP & ACTIVE SUPINATION
Hold a rolled-up towel in both hands. Use your weak hand to twist the towel in a wringing action. Repeat.

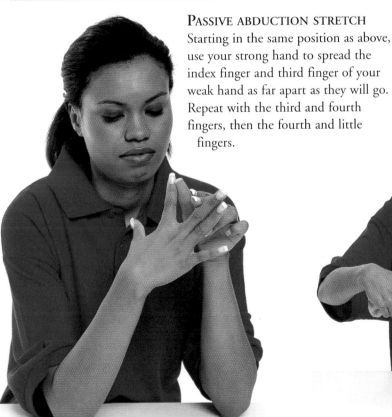

WRIST STRENGTHENING

RESISTED WRIST MOVEMENTS

1 Sitting at a table, use a soft weight to practise repeated movements to strengthen the wrist. Place your forearm flat on the table, with your hand palm up. Repeat each exercise as many times as you can.

2 Moving from the wrist, lift your hand up as far as it will go. Lower and repeat. Turn your hand over so that the palm is flat on the table. Lifting from the wrist, raise your hand as far as it will go. Lower and repeat. With palm downward and moving from the wrist only, slide your hand from side to side. Feel the pull in the sides of your wrist.

3 With fingers lightly clenched, twist your wrist and forearm back and forth so that the palm faces up, then down, then up again.

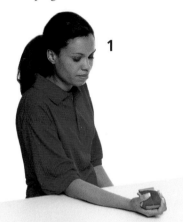
1

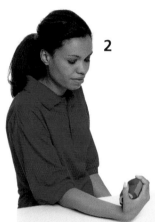
2

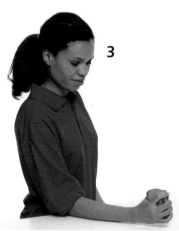
3

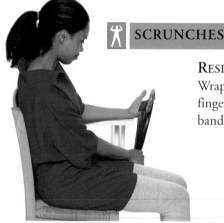

SCRUNCHES

RESISTED WRIST MOVEMENTS

Wrap an elastic exercise band round your fingers, passing one end between index finger and thumb, and repeat the exercises shown above. Hold the ends of the band firmly in your other hand so that your weak hand has to pull against it.

PRESS-UPS

WEIGHT-BEARING WRIST EXTENSION

Lie face down on the floor with your elbows bent and your hands flat on the floor and level with your shoulders. Keeping your body and legs in a straight line, straighten your arms and lift yourself off the ground so that you are balanced on hands and toes. Hold, relax and repeat.

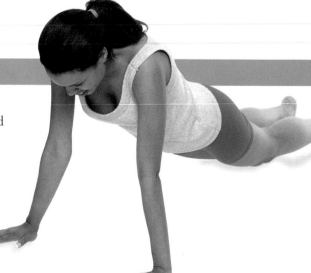

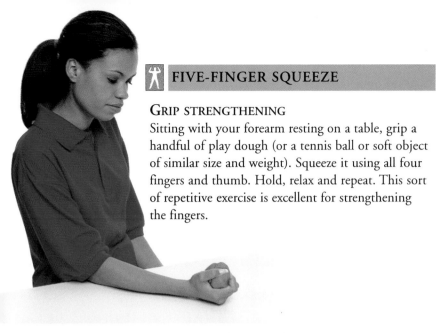

FIVE-FINGER SQUEEZE

GRIP STRENGTHENING
Sitting with your forearm resting on a table, grip a handful of play dough (or a tennis ball or soft object of similar size and weight). Squeeze it using all four fingers and thumb. Hold, relax and repeat. This sort of repetitive exercise is excellent for strengthening the fingers.

BAND STRETCH

RESISTED EXTENSION
Wrap a rubber band round your fingers and thumb. Stretch them as far apart as they will go. Feel the stretch in your fingers and thumb as they push against the band. Repeat 8 to 10 times. Move the band lower down your fingers and repeat.

SCISSOR GRIP

INTEROSSEI STRENGTHENING
1 Sitting, with your elbows bent and arms close to your sides, hold a sheet of paper between the fingers of your weak hand, keeping the fingers straight.
2 With your strong hand, try to pull the paper away, using the fingers of your weak hand to resist the pull. Alternate by moving the paper to the next two fingers, then the next, then back again.

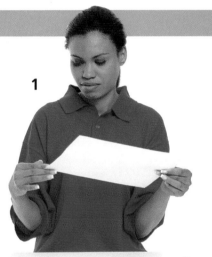

PALM SQUEEZE

FINGER & WRIST FLEXION
1 Sit with your elbow bent and forearm resting on a table, palm up.
2 Fold your fingers over and squeeze them into the palm of your hand. Hold, relax and repeat as often as you can, up to 20 times.

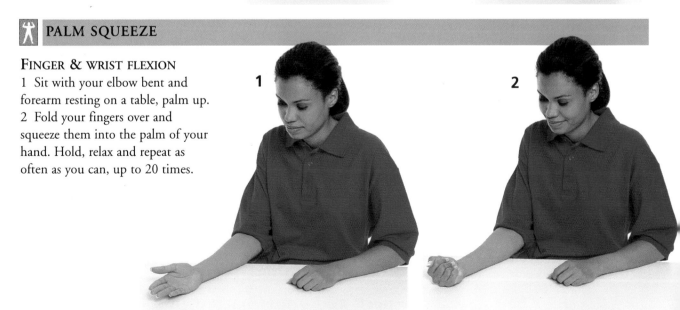

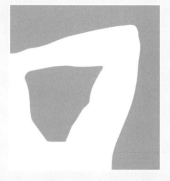

Elbow Exercises

"Tennis elbow" is quite a common problem, even in people who don't play tennis. It is a term used to describe pain around the outside of the elbow, thought to arise from repeated use of the muscles which attach to the bone nearby. It is a type of overuse injury, meaning that the tissues have had to respond to an unusual level of use. The muscles which run down the forearm to the hand are involved in gripping, so activities that require gripping – or gripping and twisting – can be painful. This can mean anything from holding a pen to wringing out a towel. At the same time, straightening the arm may be difficult, making carrying even a light shopping bag awkward. Mobility exercises are very important in the early stages of this sort of problem.

There are other reasons for elbow pain, and a person may have problems first in one elbow, then the other. Physiotherapists may also treat the neck and upper back if problems there may have precipitated the elbow pain.

HOW TO GET STARTED

• Start with the beginners' exercises for mobility. If you can do them all easily, try the beginners' exercises for flexibility, then those for strength and stability. If they are all easy, move on to the intermediate level.

• If at any stage you find an exercise is difficult – either because it hurts or because you cannot do the movement – you have identified a problem area. Work through the rest of the exercises at that level and see if any more are difficult. Repeat those particular exercises every day and you should find they become easier.

• Work on one level of exercises only. Do not attempt any at the intermediate level until you can do all the beginners' exercises comfortably. The same applies when you progress from the intermediate to the advanced level.

⚫ ELBOW BENDS

ELBOW FLEXION IN PRONATION & SUPINATION

1 Sitting, rest your forearm on a table, palm down.

2 Bend your elbow and gently lift your forearm as far as it will go without hurting, keeping your fingers and thumb relaxed. Repeat as often as is comfortable.

3 Turn your hand palm up and repeat the same exercise.

BEGINNERS' EXERCISES

The exercises in this section are the first step toward restoring mobility, flexibility, strength and stability to the elbow – both in the joint itself and in the soft tissues (muscles, tendons and ligaments) surrounding it. The movements should not hurt. If you feel pain, stop, but try to repeat the exercises a few times a day – you should soon find that your elbow moves more easily and freely.

1

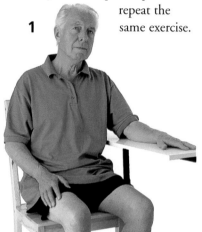

2

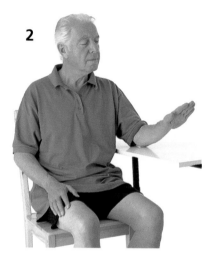

3

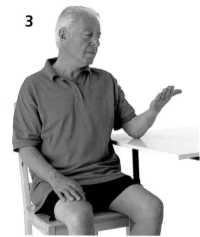

⚫ FOREARM TWIST

PRONATION & SUPINATION

Sit with your weak arm hanging loosely by your side and your palm facing in toward your chair. Place your other hand on the elbow, then use it to help twist your forearm back and forth so that your palm is facing out, then in again. Repeat as often as is comfortable.

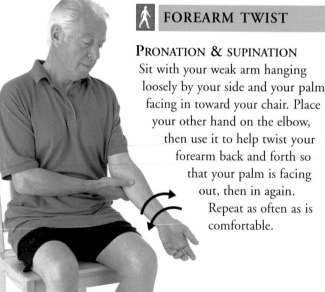

⚫ FOREARM TWIST

PRONATION & SUPINATION

Sitting at a table, rest your forearm on it with your hand on its side and thumb pointing up. Rotate your forearm so that your palm faces up; then rotate it so that your palm faces down. Repeat as often as is comfortable.

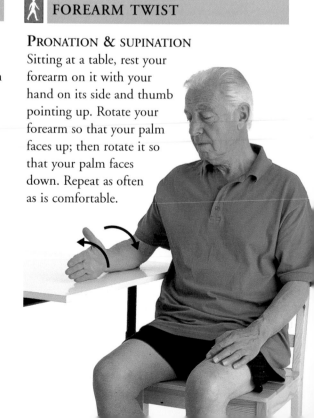

ICE THERAPY

Sitting at a table, rest your forearm on it with the palm facing upward. Place an ice pack (or cold pack) in the fold of your elbow. If your skin is sensitive, put some olive oil or baby oil on it first. Leave for about 10 minutes. This helps to reduce pain and inflammation and increase blood flow in the soft tissues around the elbow.

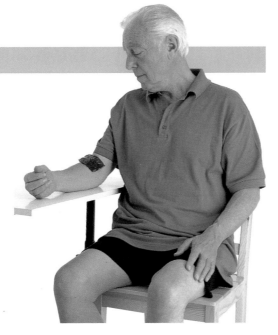

MASSAGE

Use your fingers to massage the soft tissue in the crease of your weak elbow. It may feel solid, like thick dough, but it should loosen as you work it. (Press the tissue round your strong elbow to compare how it should feel.)

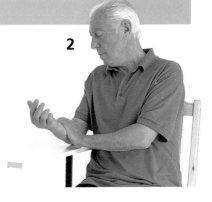

 ## FOREARM BEND

RESISTED ELBOW FLEXION

1 Sitting at a table, rest your forearm on it, with palm up and fingers relaxed. Place your other hand across your forearm.

2 Lift your forearm gently and push against the pressure exerted by the other hand. Relax and repeat.

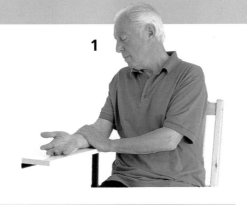

FOREARM TWIST

RESISTED ELBOW FLEXION

1 Sit at a table with your weak forearm resting on it. Start with your hand on its side and your thumb upward. Place your strong hand on your weak forearm.

2 Moving from the elbow, twist your forearm so that the palm is facing up, resisting with your strong hand. The movement should come from your elbow and wrist. Relax and repeat as often as is comfortable.

3 Return to the starting position, then twist your weak hand so that the palm is facing down, resisting with your other hand.

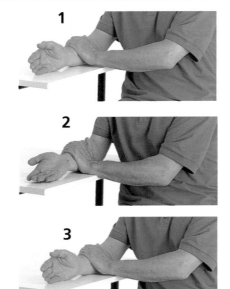

ELBOW STRETCH

RESISTED ELBOW EXTENSION

Sit with your weak elbow bent and palm up. Place the fingers of your other hand on the back of your elbow and the thumb in the crease of it. Try to straighten your weak arm, pushing against the resistance of your strong arm.

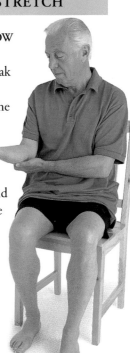

INTERMEDIATE EXERCISES

Move on to these exercises only when you can do all the beginners' ones easily and without discomfort. These require more strength and flexibility and you should be able to hold positions for longer. Repeat exercises 6–8 times unless otherwise stated.

ASSISTED ELBOW BENDS

ELBOW FLEXION WITH OVERPRESSURE IN PRONATION & SUPINATION

1 Bend your weak elbow to an angle of 90 degrees, with your palm facing up.

2 Place your other hand round your wrist and push gently to help your weak arm bend up toward the shoulder, keeping your elbow tucked in to the side of your body. Hold, relax and repeat.

3 Repeat the exercise, starting with your weak hand facing down.

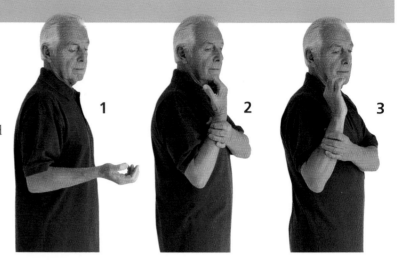

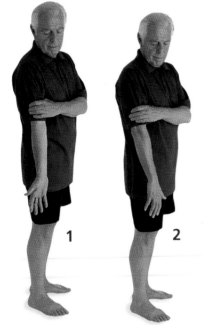

ELBOW STRAIGHTENING

PRONATION & SUPINATION IN EXTENSION

1 Stand with your weak arm hanging loosely by your side and your hand facing forward. Straighten your arm as far as is comfortable. Hold your upper arm firmly with your other hand so that it does not turn as you straighten your elbow. Hold, relax and repeat.

2 Repeat the same exercise, this time starting with your hand facing your body.

FOREARM ROTATION

PRONATION & SUPINATION IN FLEXION

1 Stand with your elbow bent at an angle of 90 degrees, your other hand cupping your elbow (or forearm, if that is more comfortable). Keep the fingers of your weak hand straight.

2 Rotate your forearm back and forth so that your palm faces first up, then down.

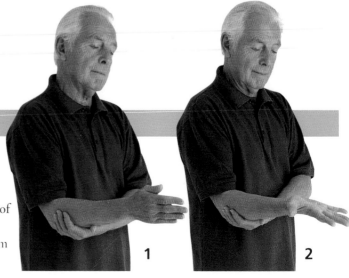

BACKWARD STRETCH

ANTERIOR STRETCH

Stand with your weak arm hanging loosely by your side. Stretch it out behind you so that your fingers are pointing backward and your thumb up toward the ceiling. Hold to feel a gentle stretch through the front of your elbow, relax and repeat.

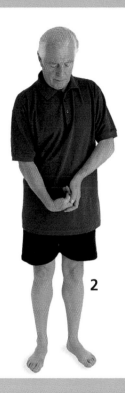

FOREARM STRETCH

EXTENSOR STRETCH

1 Stand with both arms straight down in front of you. Keeping your weak hand relaxed, cup it with your strong hand.

2 Use your strong hand to pull your weak one upward, so that you feel a gentle stretch in your weak forearm and the back of your elbow. Hold, relax and repeat.

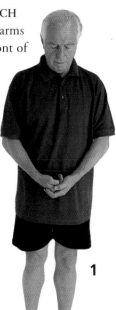

1   **2**

BENT ELBOW RAISE

POSTERIOR STRETCH

1 Stand with your weak arm hanging by your side. Bend your elbow and raise your forearm into a salute-like position slightly behind your body, with your palm facing forward and your fingers in line with your ear, spread apart and pointing backward. Hold to feel a gentle stretch. Twist your forearm forward so that your palm turns in toward your head and your thumb points backward.

2 Variation: bend your elbow so that your hand is slightly in front of your shoulder, with the fingers curled in and the back of the hand facing forward. Twist your forearm so that your palm faces forward.

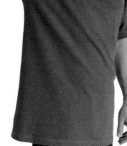

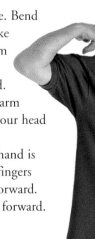

1   **2**

CONTROLLED ELBOW BENDS

1 Standing, pass a knotted elastic exercise band under the foot on your weak side and slip your hand into the other end, palm down. Keeping your elbow tucked in to your side, bend it to raise your arm as high as is comfortable. Lower it *gradually*, using your muscles to control the release. Repeat up to 20 times.
2 Repeat the same exercise with the palm of your hand facing up.
3 Repeat the same exercise with your hand side on and your thumb facing upward.
Variation: do each of the three positions in turn, repeating the sequence up to 20 times.

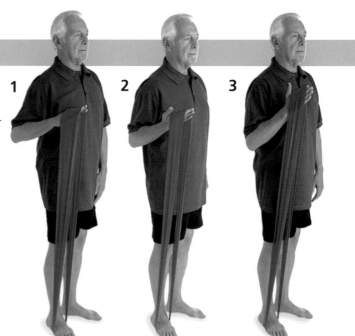

WALL PUSH-UPS

TRICEPS STRENGTHENING
With your feet about a hip's width apart and legs straight, stand at arms' length from a wall. Place your hands on the wall and bend your elbows so that you are leaning slightly forward. Slowly straighten your arms. Hold, relax and repeat.

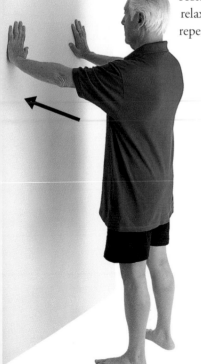

ELBOW RAISE

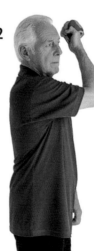

FLEXION WITH ROTATION
1 Wearing or holding a small weight, stand with your weak arm stretched out behind you and a little away from your body, palm and thumb facing backward.
2 Bend your elbow and twist your arm up and across your body in an arc, until your hand is just above your opposite shoulder, thumb pointing forward. Repeat up to 20 times.

UPWARD STRETCH

ELEVATION WITH ROTATION
1 Wearing or holding a small weight, stand with your weak arm across your body, your elbow as straight as possible and your hand on your opposite hip.
2 Twist your arm up in an arc out to your side to finish with it stretched upward, palm facing inward and thumb back, fingers and shoulder relaxed. Repeat up to 20 times.

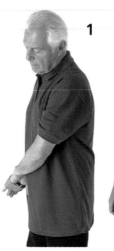

ELBOW TWIST

RESISTED FLEXION WITH PRONATION & SUPINATION

1 Wearing or holding a small weight, stand with your arm hanging down at your side, elbow slightly bent.

2 Twist your forearm in and out, while bending your elbow more and more.

3 Finish with your hand close to your opposite shoulder. Repeat the exercise the other way, twisting your forearm while straightening your elbow. Repeat the sequence as many times as you can.

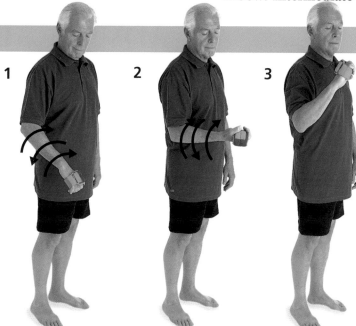

CHAIR PUSH-UPS

RESISTED EXTENSION

1 Sit on a chair, holding the seat with both hands with your elbows bent.

2 Gradually straighten your arms to lift your bottom off the chair. Your feet should be flat on the floor and you should also push up through your feet. Hold, relax and repeat.

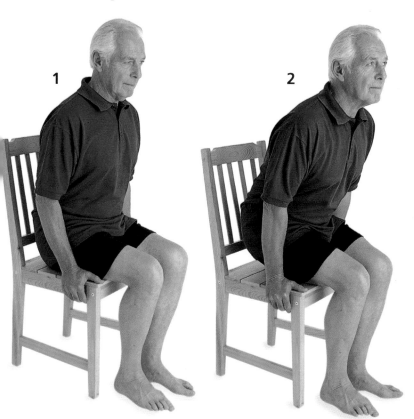

ELBOW BENDS

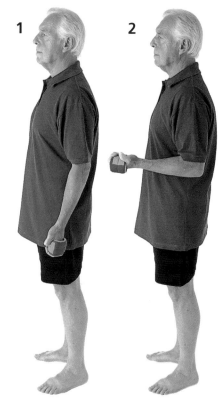

BICEPS STRENGTHENING

1 Wearing or holding a small weight, stand with your arm at your side.

2 Bend your elbow up to an angle of 90 degrees. Lower slowly, controlling the movement. Repeat up to 20 times.

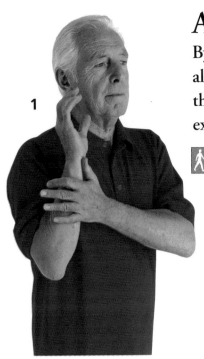

1

ADVANCED EXERCISES

By the time you reach these exercises you should have almost the full range of movement in your elbow and the soft tissues surrounding it. Repeat the strengthening exercises until fatigued.

ASSISTED ELBOW BEND

FLEXION OVERPRESSURE IN PRONATION & SUPINATION

2

1 Stand or sit with your weak elbow bent so that your hand is close to your shoulder, with the palm facing forward. Use your other hand to push against the forearm, to bring it toward your shoulder. Hold, relax and repeat.

2 Variation: repeat the same exercise starting with your palm facing your body.

ASSISTED ELBOW STRAIGHTENING

EXTENSION OVERPRESSURE

1 Standing with your weak hand resting on a table, spread the four fingers of your other hand across your weak forearm and the thumb behind your weak elbow. Use your strong hand to help your weak arm to straighten at the elbow as far as is comfortable.

2 Start in the same position, this time with the four fingers of your strong hand pointing down your forearm and the thumb behind your weak elbow. Push from behind with your thumb and from the front with your fingers.

3 Start in the same position, but hold your weak forearm with your strong hand so that the thumb is on the inner forearm. Twist your weak arm away from your body, straightening the elbow as far as is comfortable.

1

2

3

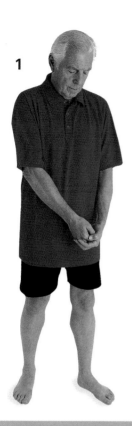

1

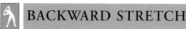

BACKWARD STRETCH

ANTERIOR STRETCH
Stand with your arm hanging loosely by your side. Stretch it out behind you so that your fingers are pointing backward and your thumb up at the ceiling. At the same time, lean your head slightly toward your strong side. Hold and feel a comfortable stretch. Repeat 2 to 3 times.

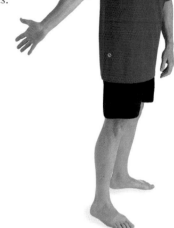

FOREARM STRETCH

EXTENSOR LENGTH
1 Stand with both arms straight in front of you, close to the hip on your strong side.
2 Keeping your weak hand relaxed, cup it with your strong hand and pull to feel a gentle stretch in your weak forearm and behind your elbow. Hold, relax and repeat.

2

BACKWARD STRETCH

POSTERIOR STRETCH
1 Stand with your weak arm hanging by your side. Bend your elbow and raise your forearm into a salute-like position slightly behind your body, with your palm facing forward and fingers relaxed in line with your ear. Tilt your head away slightly. Hold to feel a gentle stretch, relax and repeat.
2 Repeat the same exercise, but this time with your hand slightly in front of your body, your palm facing backward and fingers curled in toward your palm.

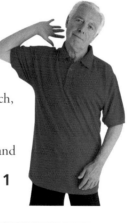

1

2

TWO-ARM BACKWARD STRETCH

AUTO-ASSISTED EXTENSION
Stand with your arms behind you, palms facing inward and fingers linked. Keeping your back and shoulders straight, straighten your elbows and lift your hands as high as is comfortable (don't worry if it is not very far). Hold, relax and repeat.

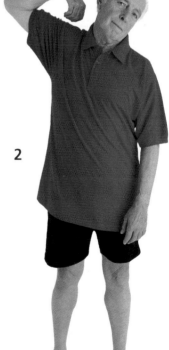

PRESS-UPS

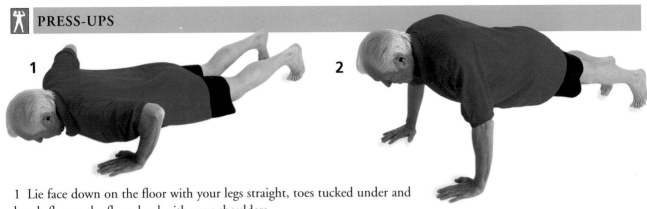

1 Lie face down on the floor with your legs straight, toes tucked under and hands flat on the floor, level with your shoulders.
2 Keeping your legs and body straight, straighten your elbows and lift yourself off the ground so that you are supported by feet and hands only. Repeat up to 20 times.

CROSS-BODY STRETCH

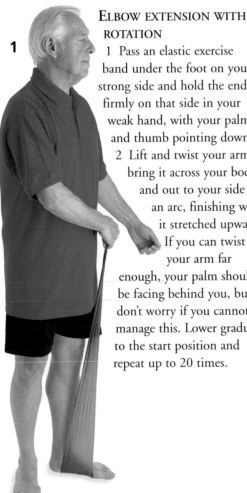

ELBOW EXTENSION WITH ROTATION

1 Pass an elastic exercise band under the foot on your strong side and hold the ends firmly on that side in your weak hand, with your palm and thumb pointing down.
2 Lift and twist your arm to bring it across your body and out to your side in an arc, finishing with it stretched upward. If you can twist your arm far enough, your palm should be facing behind you, but don't worry if you cannot manage this. Lower gradually to the start position and repeat up to 20 times.

UPWARD STRETCH

ELBOW FLEXION WITH ROTATION

1 Pass an elastic exercise band under the foot on your weak side and hold the ends firmly in the hand on the same side. Stand with your arm behind you and a little away from your body, your palm facing out to the side.
2 Bend your elbow to bring your arm up and across your body in an arc, ending up with your hand above your opposite shoulder. Lower gradually to the start position and repeat up to 20 times.

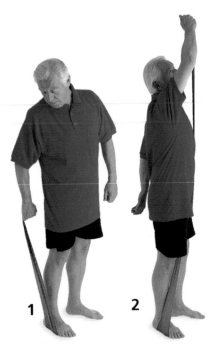

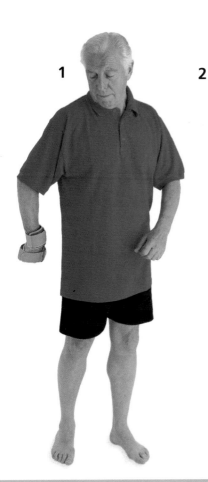

CROSS-BODY STRETCH

1 Wearing a hand weight around the wrist on your weak side and holding another one in the same hand, stand with your arm stretched out behind you and a little away from your body, your palm facing backward.

2 Bend your elbow to bring your arm up and across your body in an arc, finishing with your hand just above your opposite shoulder, the thumb pointing behind your ear. Then return your arm to the starting position, controlling the weight smoothly as you lower it. Repeat up to 20 times.

RESISTED ELBOW BEND

RESISTED ELBOW FLEXION/EXTENSION

1 Standing, pass a knotted elastic exercise band under the foot on your weak side and slip your hand into the other end, palm upward and fingers closed. Keeping your arm tucked in to your side, bend your elbow to raise your arm as high as is comfortable. Lower it gradually, using your muscles to control the release. Repeat up to 20 times.

2 Repeat the same exercise with your palm facing the floor.

3 Repeat the same exercise with your palm facing in toward your mid-line and your thumb pointing upward.

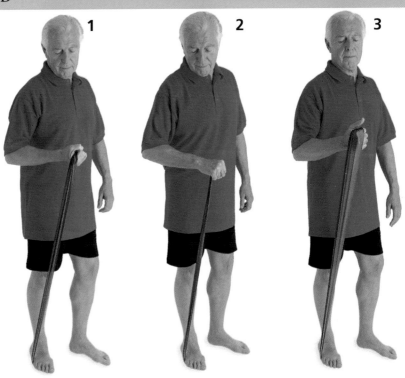

Shoulder Exercises

A healthy shoulder joint allows a great deal of mobility. It is a ball and socket joint, but the socket is so shallow that it is almost flat, which is why the shoulder can normally move so freely. It is surrounded by a complex of muscles (the rotator cuff) which are finely tuned to work together and support the joint. There is great scope for injury around the shoulder: the muscles may be torn, the ligaments or tendons irritated, the shoulder itself dislocated or the bones fractured.

Depending on the nature of your problem, you may find a certain movement – such as lifting your arm above your head – difficult and painful, or you may find that all the movement in the joint is restricted.

The exercises in this chapter address all these problems and, as you work through them, you should be able to identify those that are most therapeutic for your particular injury.

HOW TO GET STARTED

• Start with the beginners' exercises for mobility. If you can do them all easily, try the beginners' exercises for flexibility, then those for strength and stability. If they are all easy, move on to the intermediate level.

• If at any stage you find an exercise is difficult – either because it hurts or because you cannot do the movement – you have identified a problem area. Work through the rest of the exercises at that level and see if any more are difficult. Repeat those particular exercises every day and you should find it becomes easier.

• Work on one level of exercises only. Do not attempt any at the intermediate level until you can do all the beginners' exercises comfortably. The same applies when you progress from the intermediate to the advanced level.

MOBILITY

BEGINNER
Shoulder stretch	84
Pendular movements	84
Assisted shoulder lifts	85

INTERMEDIATE
Back reach	88
Wall crawl	88
Cross-body stretch	88
Elbow glide	89
Arm raise	89
Sideways push	89
Backward stretch	89

ADVANCED
Upward stretches	93
Overhead reach	93

FLEXIBILITY

BEGINNER
Shoulder-blade control	86
Shoulder stretch	86

INTERMEDIATE
Shoulder stability	90
Backward stretch	90
Shoulder stretch	90
Pendular movements	90
Upward stretch	90
Weight bearing	91
Upper arm stretch	91
Underarm stretch	91
Underarm stretch	92

ADVANCED
Overhead stretch	94
Cross-body stretch	94
Long stretch	94
Side stretch	94

STRENGTH & STABILITY

BEGINNER
Shoulder rotation	87
Shoulder strength	87
Shoulder roll	87

INTERMEDIATE
Weight bearing	92
Upper arm rotation	92

ADVANCED
Overhead cross stretch	94
Shoulder-blade control	94
Resisted scrunches	95
Sideways rotation	96
Diagonal scrunches	96
Upward & crossways lifts	96
Inward scrunch	97
Triceps strength	97
Arm lift	97
Shoulder circling	97

BEGINNERS' EXERCISES

These exercises are the first step towards restoring
mobility, flexibility, and strength and
stability to the shoulder. Repeat each
exercise only as often as is comfortable.

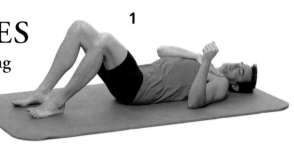

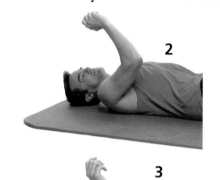

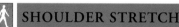

SHOULDER STRETCH

1 Lie on your back with your legs either straight or bent, whichever is more
comfortable. Keeping your weak upper arm close to your body, bend your
elbow to an angle of 90 degrees so that your forearm sticks up in the air.
2 Lift your elbow off the floor as far as is comfortable, keeping it close to
your body. Hold, then lower your elbow to the floor again.
3 Slide your elbow away from your body to an angle of about 45 degrees.
Hold, then return to the starting position.
4 Roll your forearm away from your body as far as is comfortable. Hold.
5 Roll your arm in across your stomach. Hold.
6 Raise your arm with elbow bent and stretch your forearm straight across
the top of your body so that your hand rests on your opposite shoulder.
Hold, relax and repeat the whole sequence.

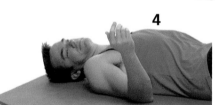

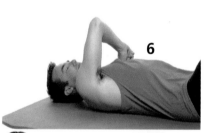

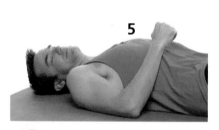

PENDULAR MOVEMENTS

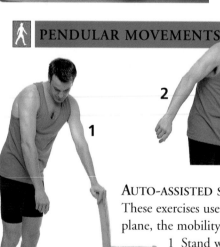

AUTO-ASSISTED SHOULDER MOBILITY
These exercises use the weight of the arm like a pendulum so that as the arm gently swings in each
plane, the mobility at the shoulder joint gradually increases.
1 Stand with your strong arm resting on a chair, your weak arm relaxed at your side.
2 Let the weak arm swing behind you and back again with the palm facing your body.
3 Bring your arm forward and across the front of your body to the opposite hip. Repeat.
4 Let your arm swing out in front of you as far as it will go comfortably (it may not be
very far). Repeat.
5 Then stretch it out behind you. Relax and repeat the whole sequence.

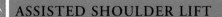

ASSISTED SHOULDER LIFT

AUTO-ASSISTED GLENO-HUMERAL FLEXION
Stand with your arms straight out in front of you,
hands loosely clasped. Keeping your elbows straight, lift
your hands gently, using the strength of the strong arm
to help raise the weak one.

ASSISTED SHOULDER LIFT

GLENO-HUMERAL FLEXION
1 Standing, hold a walking stick or broom handle with both hands.
Start with your arms by your side.
2 Gently bend your elbows and raise your hands until they are level
with your shoulders (or as far as they will go comfortably).
3 Straighten your elbows and hold the stick at about the level of your
shoulders.

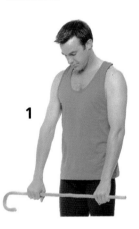

1

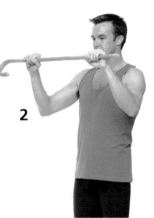

2

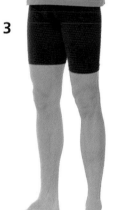

3

ASSISTED SHOULDER LIFT

HORIZONTAL ABDUCTION & ADDUCTION
1 Holding a walking stick or broom handle as above,
straighten your arms and hold the stick away from your
body, at about waist height.
2 Keeping your arms straight and moving from the
shoulders, not the waist, move the stick round to your left.
Hold, relax, then move it to your right as far as is
comfortable. Hold, relax and repeat. Your
strong arm will help the weaker one.

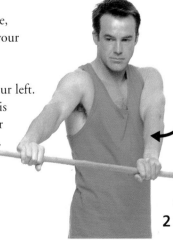

1

2

SHOULDER-BLADE CONTROL

SCAPULAR STABILITY

Stand with your back to a wall, your feet slightly away from it, knees slightly bent and bottom resting against the wall. Let your arms rest by your sides or clasp your hands loosely in front of you. Pull your stomach up and in and push your shoulder blades against the wall. Hold, relax and repeat. This exercise strengthens the muscles around the shoulder blades.

SHOULDER STRETCH

AUTO-ASSISTED HORIZONTAL FLEXION & EXTENSION

1 Standing, fold your arms so that your strong hand is supporting your weak elbow on the weak side at about waist level.

2 Lift your arms so that they are straight out in front of you. Use your strong arm to help.

3 Moving from the shoulders, not the waist, twist your arms round to the left.

4 Relax, then twist them to the right. Relax and repeat.

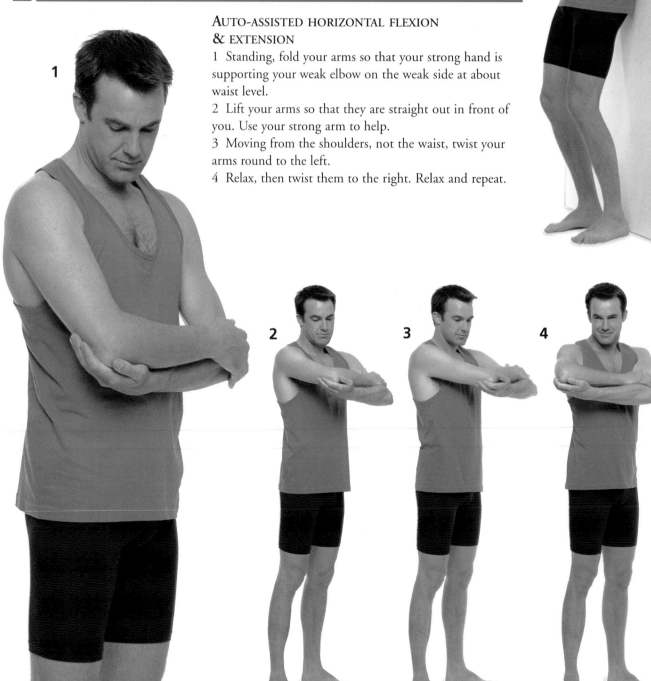

🏃 SHOULDER ROTATION

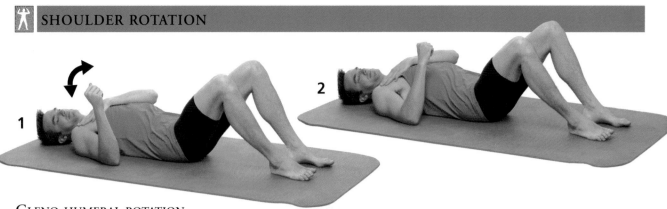

GLENO-HUMERAL ROTATION

1 Lie on your back on the floor with your upper arm at an angle of about 45 degrees to your body, your elbow bent and your forearm sticking up in the air. Put your other hand on your weak shoulder to feel the movement. Gently roll your forearm away from your body toward the floor.

2 Relax, then roll your arm in toward your ribcage. Relax and repeat up to 30 times.

🏃 SHOULDER STRENGTH

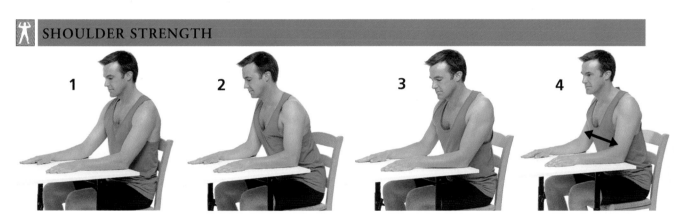

PARTIAL WEIGHT-BEARING PROPRIOCEPTION

1 Sit with your hands and forearms on a table, elbows bent.

2 Lean slightly forward on to your elbows, pushing down on your forearms. Take as much weight as possible on your weak arm. Relax.

3 From the same position lean slightly to the right, again taking as much weight as possible on your weak arm.

4 Then lean slightly to the left. Relax and repeat.

🏃 SHOULDER ROLL

LOWER TRAPEZIUS

Sitting upright in a chair, rotate both shoulders back in an arc, working the muscles around the shoulder blades. Hold at the backward point of the arc for 10 seconds, then relax and repeat.

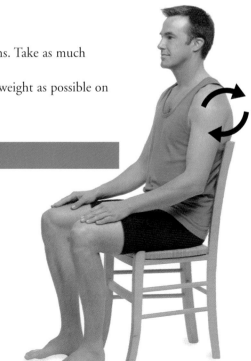

INTERMEDIATE EXERCISES

Do not attempt these exercises until you can do all the beginners' exercises comfortably. Your shoulder should be stronger and more mobile than when you began, and the soft tissues should be stronger. Unless otherwise stated, repeat each exercise 6 to 8 times.

 WALL CRAWL

ASSISTED FLEXION
Stand with your forearm resting against a wall. Gradually slide your arm up the wall using a "creeping" movement of your fingers. This exercise increases mobility in the shoulder.

CROSS-BODY STRETCH

HORIZONTAL FLEXION
Stand with your arms relaxed by your side. Raise your weak arm and bend your elbow at shoulder height to bring your hand across your chest as far as it will go toward the opposite shoulder. This exercise increases mobility in the shoulder. You should feel a stretch on the outside of your upper arm.

 BACK REACH

AUTO-ASSISTED EXTENSION & MEDIAL ROTATION
Stand with your weak hand clasping the end of a rolled-up towel behind your back at about waist level and your strong hand clasping the other end behind your neck. Move your arms down (1) and up (2) as if you were drying your back.
This exercise increases mobility in the shoulder.

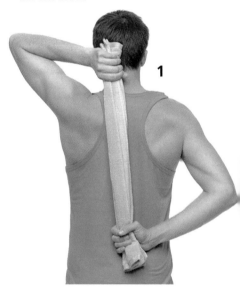

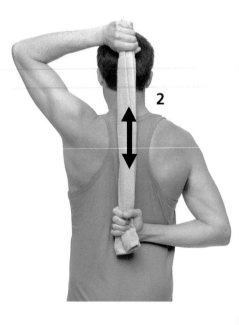

ELBOW GLIDE

INFERIOR GLIDE

Sit at a table with your weak forearm resting on it, elbow bent. With your other hand, press down gently on the point of your shoulder. Keeping your hand on the table, lift your elbow up and slightly away from your body. Hold, relax and repeat.

This exercise increases mobility between the joint surfaces in the shoulder.

ARM RAISE

ASSISTED FLEXION

1 Standing, hold a walking stick or broom handle in both hands. Start with your arms straight down in front of you.
2 Keeping your arms straight, raise the stick as high as you can above your head, then lower it and repeat.

This strengthens the shoulder muscles and increases mobility. You will probably find that the muscles tire quite quickly.

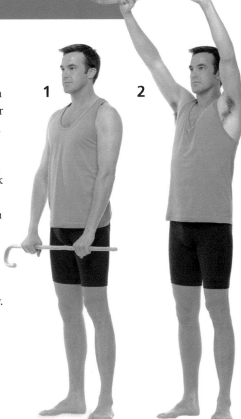

SIDEWAYS PUSH

LATERAL DISTRACTION

Sit at a table with your weak forearm resting on it, elbow bent. Place your other hand round your upper arm, with the thumb close to your armpit. Move your arm in toward your body, pushing against the pressure of your thumb.

BACKWARD STRETCH

POSTERIOR GLIDE

Sit with your back to a table and your weak arm stretched out behind you with the hand flat on the table. Put your other hand on your shoulder and use light pressure on the shoulder joint as you twist your body slightly away (i.e. to the left if your injury is to the right shoulder and vice versa).

This exercise increases mobility between the joint surfaces in the shoulder.

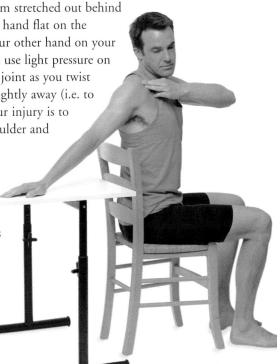

SHOULDER STABILITY

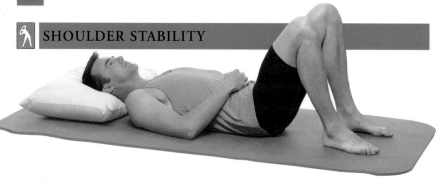

Lie on your back on the floor with a pillow under your head and your hands clasped loosely over your stomach. Push your shoulders back into the floor, working the muscles around your shoulder blades. Hold, relax and repeat.

SHOULDER STRETCH

SHOULDER FLEXION

1 Lie on your back on the floor with a pillow or cushion under your head. With your weak upper arm close to your body, bend your elbow so that your forearm points up in the air.

2 Keeping your elbow bent, raise your upper arm so that your hand touches the pillow above your head. Hold, relax and repeat.

PENDULAR MOVEMENTS

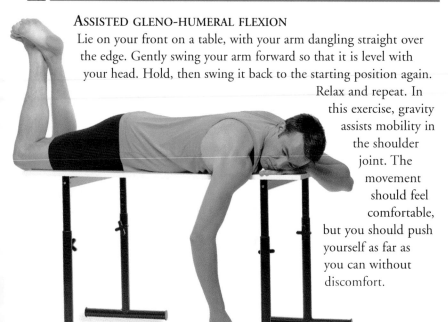

ASSISTED GLENO-HUMERAL FLEXION

Lie on your front on a table, with your arm dangling straight over the edge. Gently swing your arm forward so that it is level with your head. Hold, then swing it back to the starting position again. Relax and repeat. In this exercise, gravity assists mobility in the shoulder joint. The movement should feel comfortable, but you should push yourself as far as you can without discomfort.

BACKWARD STRETCH

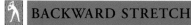

ANTERIOR FLEXIBILITY

Standing, stretch your arm straight out behind you, palm facing forward, fingers straight and thumb pointing back, away from the fingers. Hold, relax and repeat.

UPWARD STRETCH

SHOULDER FLEXION

Stand facing a wall, bend your weak arm and rest your elbow on the wall. Stretch your hand back over your shoulder and feel the stretch under your arm. Hold, relax and repeat.

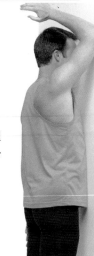

WEIGHT BEARING

PROPRIOCEPTION IN FLEXION

Lie face down on the floor with your elbows bent and your forearms and hands flat on the floor. Your elbows should be about level with your shoulders. Without moving your hands or forearms, raise your chest off the floor and concentrate on the weight going through your arms to the floor. Hold, relax and repeat.

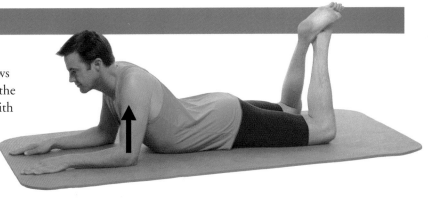

UPPER ARM STRETCH

SCAPULO-HUMERAL FLEXIBILITY

Sit facing a table, with your weak arm stretched out on the table in front of you. Bend forward from the waist so that most of the arm is resting on the table. Hold, feeling the stretch under your arm. Relax and repeat.

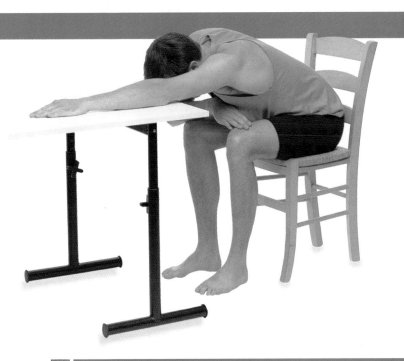

UNDERARM STRETCH

INFERIOR GLIDE

Sit on a table, close to one end so that you can comfortably grip the edge of the table to your weak side. Lean gently away, to feel a stretch under your arm. Hold, relax and repeat.

WEIGHT BEARING

PROPRIOCEPTION IN EXTENSION

Lie on your back with your knees bent and prop yourself up on your elbows so that your head and shoulders are raised and your elbows and forearms flat on the floor. Hold this position for 10 to 20 seconds.

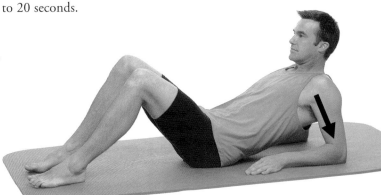

WEIGHT BEARING

Proprioception in kneeling

1 Kneel with your hands directly under your shoulders and flat on the floor. Without moving your hands or knees, lean your body forward. Hold, relax and repeat.
2 Then lean back, hold, relax and repeat.

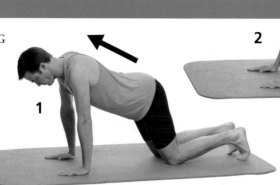

WEIGHT BEARING

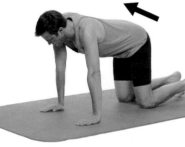

Proprioception in kneeling

Kneel with your hands directly under your shoulders and flat on the floor. Without moving your hands or knees, lean to the right, hold your balance, then lean to the left and hold. Relax and repeat.

UPPER ARM ROTATION

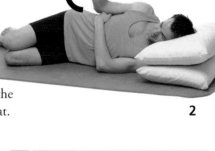

1 Lie on your side with your weak arm uppermost. Hold or wear a small weight. Keep your upper arm close to your body and bend your elbow at an angle of 90 degrees so that your forearm and hand stick out in front of you.
2 Lift your forearm, describing an arc with your hand and taking it as far as is comfortable. Hold. Then bring your hand slowly back to the starting position. Hold, relax and repeat.

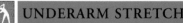

UPPER ARM ROTATION

Gleno-humeral rotation

1 Lie on your front on a table with your weak upper arm resting on it and the forearm dangling over the edge. Place a folded towel under your arm if it feels more comfortable. Keep your elbow bent at 90 degrees.
2 Slowly swing your forearm forward, hold, then return to the starting position and relax. Swing your arm back, hold and return to the starting position. Repeat the whole exercise up to 20 times.

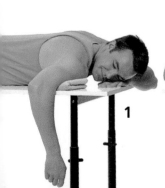

UNDERARM STRETCH

Anterior stretch

Stand with your weak arm close to your side, hand facing forward and elbow straight. Stretch your arm straight out behind you, lifting the thumb away from the fingers. Hold, relax and repeat.

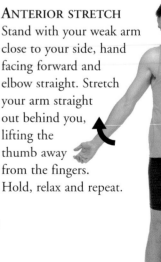

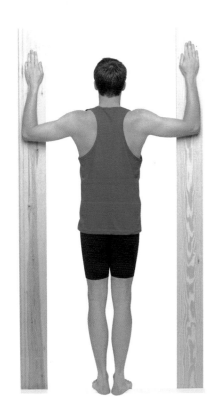

ADVANCED EXERCISES

By the time you progress to this section, your shoulder should be able to achieve almost the full range of movement. With these exercises you should feel greater stretch without discomfort or pain. Repeat the strengthening exercises until fatigued.

 UPWARD STRETCH

LOWER TRAPEZIUS

Stand in a doorway with your elbows bent, your upper arms at about shoulder level and your hands flat on the door uprights, with your fingers just above your head. Without moving your arms, pull your shoulder blades back and down. Hold, relax and repeat.

UPWARD STRETCH

SCAPULO-HUMERAL CONTROL

Standing with your back to a wall, bend your elbows to an angle of 90 degrees and slide your forearms above your head. Hold, relax and repeat.

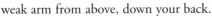 **OVERHEAD REACH**

ASSISTED EXTENSION/ADDUCTION/MEDIAL ROTATION

1 Hold a rolled-up towel behind your back, with your weak hand holding one end halfway up your back and your strong hand holding the other above your head. Move the towel up and down as if you were drying your back, assisting the reach up.

2 Change hands, putting your weak hand behind your neck and your strong one in the small of your back. Repeat the "drying" motion to assist the reach of your weak arm from above, down your back.

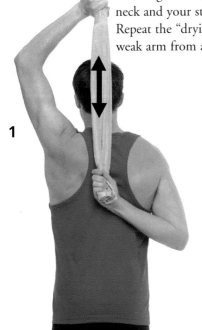

1

2

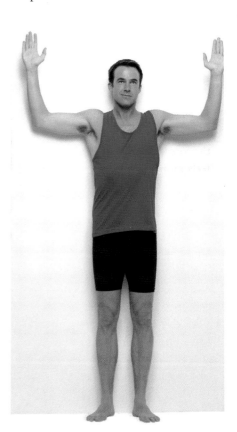

OVERHEAD STRETCH

Stand with
your arms
above your
head and place
your strong hand
on your weak
elbow. Push down
gently to help
your weak arm
reach down your
back. Hold, and
feel a stretch in
your upper arm.

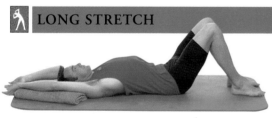

OVERHEAD CROSS STRETCH

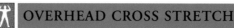

**GLENO-HUMERAL ELEVATION &
HORIZONTAL FLEXION**
In the same position, draw your weak elbow across
toward the opposite shoulder. Hold, relax and repeat.

CROSS-BODY STRETCH

**HORIZONTAL FLEXION WITH
OVERPRESSURE**
With your strong hand on the elbow
of your weak arm, bring that arm
across your body toward the other
shoulder. Hold, relax and repeat.

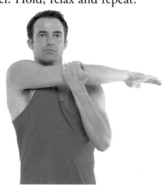

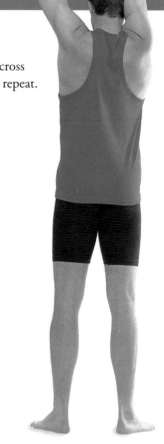

LONG STRETCH

Lie on your back with
your stomach held in.
Stretch both arms as far as
you can above your head,
palms up, aiming to rest
the backs of your hands on the floor. Hold, relax and repeat. If the small of
your back lifts off the floor, use rolled-up towels to support your arms.

SIDE STRETCH

SHOULDER-BLADE CONTROL

SCAPULAR STABILITY
1 Stand facing a wall with
your hand flat against it
and the shoulder blade on
your weak side pressing
against your index finger.
2 Move your hand up the
wall a little, maintaining
the contact between
shoulder blade and finger.

1 **2**

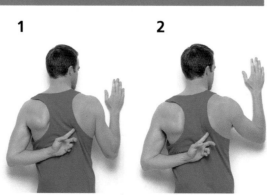

ANTERIOR FLEXIBILITY
Stand with your weak arm straight
out to the side and slightly behind
you. Keep your fingers straight and
point the thumb back. Tilt your
head gently toward the other
shoulder. Hold, relax and repeat.

RESISTED SCRUNCHES

Repeat each stage of this exercise up to 30 times. Sitting, wrap an elastic exercise band round your hand, passing it between fingers and thumb. Rest the side of your hand on a table with thumb pointing up. Hold the ends of the band in your other hand on your opposite hip (1). Keeping that hand still, pull your weak hand away from you. Slowly return to the start position (2). Repeat.

Move your strong hand to just above the knee of your weak side (3) and, keeping the hand holding the ends of the band still, lift your forearm off the table, away from you and backward (4). Slowly return to the start position. Repeat.

Ask someone else to hold the ends of the band, or tie them round the banisters. Start with your hand by your shoulder (5). Pull down against the band (6). Slowly return to the start position. Repeat.

With your forearm resting on the table, elbow bent and hand on its side, get someone else to hold the ends of the band or tie it to the table leg (7). Pull against the band, bringing your hand closer to your body (8). Slowly return to the start position. Repeat.

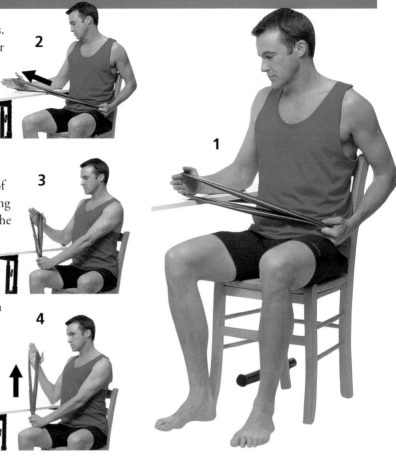

2

3

4

5 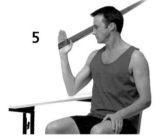 **6** 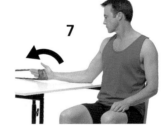 **7** 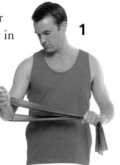 **8**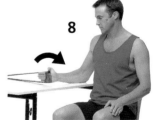

RESISTED SCRUNCHES

1 Standing, wrap an elastic exercise band round your weak arm just above the elbow. Hold the ends firmly in your other hand at waist level. With your upper arm slightly away from your body, bend your elbow so that your forearm points forward.

2 Pull against the band to take your elbow away from your side as far as it will go. Hold and repeat up to 30 times.

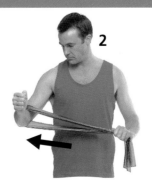

1

2

SIDEWAYS ROTATION

Wrap an elastic exercise band around your weak fingers. Keeping your upper arm close to your body, bend your elbow so that your forearm is in front of you. Hold the ends of the band firmly in your other hand by the hip on your strong side. Keeping your elbow close to your body, draw an arc with your hand pulling against the band. Slowly return and repeat as often as you can.

DIAGONAL SCRUNCHES

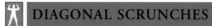

1 Standing, pass an elastic exercise band under the foot on your strong side. With your elbow bent, hold the ends in your weak hand close to your body in front of the opposite hip. The band should be just taut.
2 Lift your arm, twisting hand and forearm as they rise so that your arm is straight up above your head with your thumb pointing backward. Slowly return to the start position and repeat as often as you can.
Variation: transfer the band to the foot on your weak side and hold it in your weak hand with your thumb facing backward. Draw your hand across to the opposite hip. Straighten your arm above your head. Slowly return and repeat.

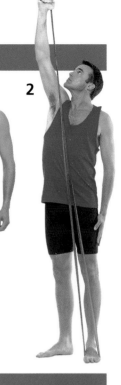

UPWARD & CROSSWAYS LIFT

SHOULDER EXTENSION WITH ROTATION

1 Fix the band to a point behind your strong shoulder, or get someone to hold it for you. Grip the other end in your weak fist, close to your head on your strong side, with thumb pointing upward.
2 Twist your arm as you straighten your elbow to pull the band down toward your opposite hip.
3 Draw the band across your body and finish with thumb pointing backward. Slowly return to the start position. Repeat as often as you can.

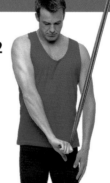
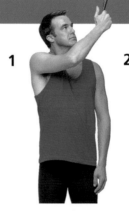
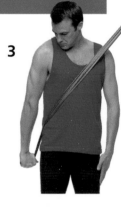

UPWARD & CROSSWAYS LIFT

RESISTED FLEXION/EXTENSION WITH ROTATION

Stand, wearing a wrist weight and/or clasping a weight loosely in your weak hand. Raise your arm straight up above your head, thumb facing backward (1). Keeping your elbow straight, gradually lower your arm, twisting as you go, so that your hand is level with the opposite shoulder and the thumb points downward (2). Continue to lower your arm until the hand is level with the opposite hip (3). Variation: start with your arm reaching across your body, and over the opposite shoulder (4). Bend elbow and twist arm across your body (5) to stretch out behind you with the thumb pointing back (6). Slowly return and repeat until fatigued.

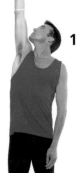
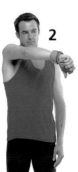
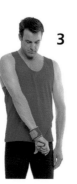
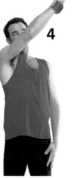
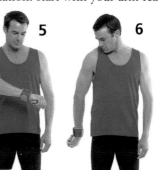

INWARD SCRUNCH

1 **RESISTED MEDIAL ROTATION**
1 Fix the ends of an elastic exercise band to the banisters or get someone else to hold them for you. Standing, place your fingers in the loop of the band. Start with your elbow close to your body, bent at an angle of 90 degrees so that your hand faces forward.
2 2 Pulling against the band and without moving your body, draw your arm across your body as far as it will go. Hold, slowly return to the start position and repeat.

ARM LIFT

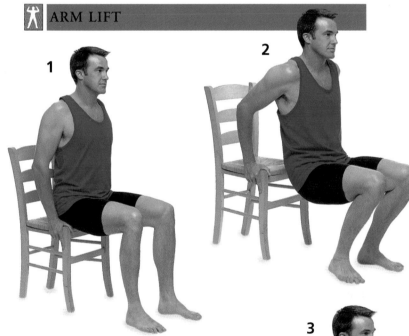

1
2
3

1 Sit on the edge of a chair with your feet flat on the floor. Grip the edge of the chair with both hands.
2 Using your arms, push forward and lift yourself off the chair.
3 Use your arms to lower you: bend your elbows at an angle of 90 degrees and lower your bottom toward the floor. Hold, slowly return to the start position and repeat.

TRICEPS STRENGTH

Standing, wrap an elastic exercise band round your weak hand, between thumb and index finger. Pass it behind your shoulders and hold the ends firmly in your other hand (or attach them to the banisters). Bend your weak elbow so that your hand is level with your shoulder. Using a slow punching motion, pull against the band and stretch your arm straight out in front of you. Hold, slowly return to the start position and repeat.

SHOULDER CIRCLING

Wearing or holding a weight, stand with your arm out to the side at

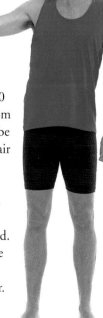

an angle of about 80 degrees. Moving from the shoulder, describe small circles in the air with your hand forward, then backward, then in a figure of eight. Repeat until fatigued. This strengthens the stabilising muscles around the shoulder.

Neck Exercises

The neck consists of a series of interlocking blocks (vertebrae), each linked on either side by a facet joint, and all but the top two separated by a disc. Problems can arise with any of these structures: it is possible to have a painful, stiff facet joint on one side only or on both sides, or pain at more than one facet joint on one or both sides, or at one or more facet joints and discs. Pain may be localized, or it may restrict a number of different movements. The exercises are designed to cover any of these problems and you will find that some are particularly appropriate for your condition. It may be necessary to work very gently and cautiously; if in doubt, seek guidance from a professional.

Warning None of the positions should be held for more than 2 to 3 seconds, particularly backward bending and/or turning. Never practise head circling.

HOW TO GET STARTED

• Start with the beginners' exercises for mobility. If you can do them all easily, try the beginners' exercises for flexibility, then those for strength and stability. If they are all easy, move on to the intermediate level.

• If at any stage you find an exercise is difficult – either because it hurts or because you cannot do the movement – you have identified a problem area. Work through the rest of the exercises at that level and see if any more are difficult. Repeat those particular exercises every day and you should find they become easier.

• Work on one level of exercises only. Do not attempt any at the intermediate level until you can do all the beginners' exercises comfortably. The same applies when you progress from the intermediate to the advanced level.

MOBILITY	
BEGINNER	
Neck turns	100
Neck tilts	100
Neck stretches	100
Nodding	102
Tipping	102
Head tilts	102
INTERMEDIATE	
Backward bend	104
Forward bend	104
Head tilts	104
Head turns	104
ADVANCED	
Backward bend	108
Forward bends	108
Head tilts	108
Head turns	108
Backward bend	109

FLEXIBILITY	
BEGINNER	
Side twists	101
Shoulder circles	101
Neck & arm stretch	101
INTERMEDIATE	
Head tilts	105
Backward bend	105
Head turns	105
Back pivot	106
Side twists	106
Backward stretch	106
Assisted pivot	107
Assisted side pivot	107
Assisted neck tilts	107
ADVANCED	
Backward stretch	109
Head tilts	109

STRENGTH & STABILITY	
BEGINNER	
Mini turns	102
Sideways tilt	103
Neck twist	103
Backward lean	103
Forward lean	103
Nodding	103
INTERMEDIATE	
Postural retraining	106
Neck scrunch	107
ADVANCED	
Neck bends	110
Head raises	110
Lower neck stretches	111
Twist ups	111

BEGINNERS' EXERCISES

These gentle exercises aim to reintroduce mobility in all directions in the neck, while encouraging muscle control and flexibility in the soft tissues. Do not do any exercise so vigorously or so often that it hurts.

NECK TURNS

NON-WEIGHT-BEARING ROTATION

1 Lie on your back with a pillow under your head. Gently turn your head to the right and return. Repeat.
2 Gently turn your head to the left and return. Repeat.

NECK TILTS

NON-WEIGHT-BEARING SIDE FLEXION

1 Lie on your back with a pillow under your head. Gently tilt your head sideways to the right, bringing your ear to your shoulder. Return and repeat.
2 Gently tilt your head sideways to the left, bringing your ear to your shoulder. Return and repeat.

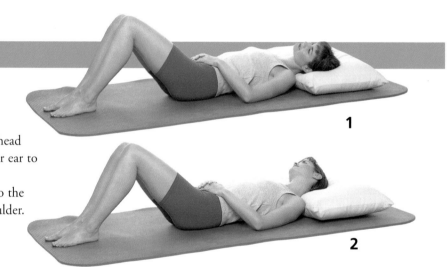

NECK STRETCHES

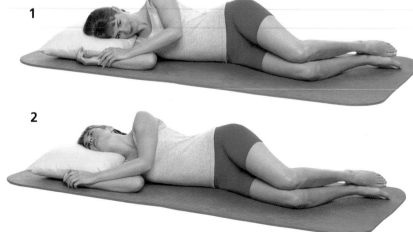

NON-WEIGHT-BEARING EXTENSION

1 Lie on whichever side is more comfortable, with a pillow under your head. Bend your head down toward your chest. Return and repeat.
2 Tip your head back gently, without letting your chin point up – i.e. keep your neck straight, don't twist it. Return and repeat.

SIDE TWISTS

Lie on whichever side is more comfortable, with a pillow under your head (1). Breathing in, gently twist your neck and lift your head slightly off the pillow (2); as you breathe out, slowly relax back down on to the pillow and stay there for 10 seconds, relaxing and breathing gently. Repeat three times.

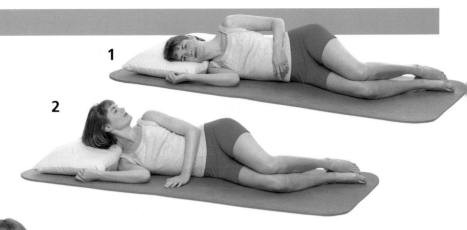

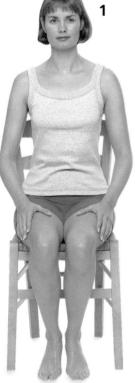

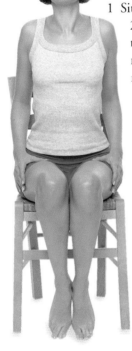

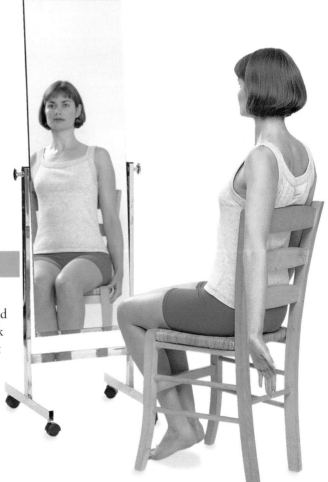 ## SHOULDER CIRCLES

1 Sit in a chair with your head and neck in a neutral, relaxed position. 2 Bring your shoulders forward and up, circling from the front to the back. Repeat a few times in a continuous movement, then reverse the movement. This relaxes the muscles which run from the neck to the shoulder.

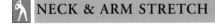 ## NECK & ARM STRETCH

Sit in front of a mirror with the arm on your weak side hanging down toward the floor, palm facing forward and hand relaxed but open. Keeping your shoulder and neck relaxed, move your arm slightly behind you, and raise it to an angle of about 45 degrees from your body. Keep your neck in a "neutral" position. Hold, relax and repeat. This mobilizes the soft tissues which run from the neck to the shoulder.

NODDING

UPPER NECK FLEXION

1 Sitting on a chair, bend both arms to bring your fingertips behind your ears. Place the tips of your index and middle fingers on the top of your neck and the base of your skull respectively, on either side. Place your thumbs on your jaw.

2 Keeping your neck still, nod your head down slightly so that the gap between your fingertips widens. Bring your head up and repeat the movement. This increases mobility at the top of the neck and its junction with the skull.

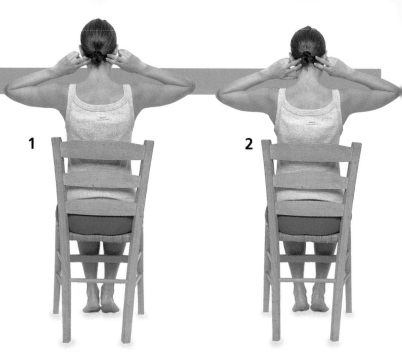

TIPPING

UPPER NECK EXTENSION

Sitting on a chair, bend both arms to bring your fingertips behind your ears. Place the tips of your index and middle fingers on the top of your neck and the base of your skull respectively; place your thumbs on your jaw. Supporting the weight of your head on your hands, gently tip your head back. Bring your head forward and repeat the movement. This increases mobility at the top of the neck and its junction with the skull.

MINI TURNS

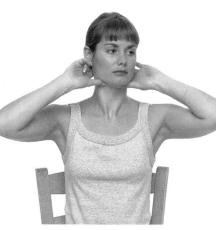

UPPER NECK ROTATION

Sitting on a chair, bend both arms to bring your fingertips behind your ears. Place the tips of your index and middle fingers on the top of your neck and the base of your skull respectively; place your thumbs on your jaw. Gently turn your head to the left, return and repeat the movement.
Variation: turn your head to the right, return and repeat the movement.

HEAD TILTS

UPPER NECK SIDE FLEXION

Sitting on a chair, bend both arms to bring your fingertips behind your ears. Place the tips of your index and middle fingers on the top of your neck and the base of your skull respectively, on either side of your spine; place your thumbs on your jaw. Keeping your shoulders level, gently tilt your head to the left, relax and repeat. Repeat the same exercise, tilting your head to the right. Relax and repeat.
Variation: do the exercise on both sides, moving your head alternately to right and left.

SIDEWAYS TILT

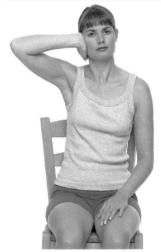

RESISTED SIDE FLEXION
Sitting on a chair, bend one arm, with your elbow pointing outward and your palm against the side of your head. Keeping your head facing forward, push your head into your hand and vice versa, so that your head does not move. Hold for 2 to 3 seconds, relax and repeat. Your physiotherapist may recommend you to do this exercise on one side only.

NECK TWIST

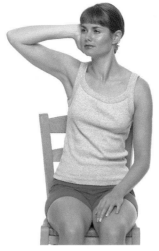

RESISTED ROTATION
Sitting on a chair, bend one arm, with your elbow pointing outward and your palm against the side of your head. Turn your head into your hand, using gentle hand pressure to resist the movement. Hold for 2 to 3 seconds, relax and repeat. Your physiotherapist may recommend you to do this exercise on one side only.

BACKWARD LEAN

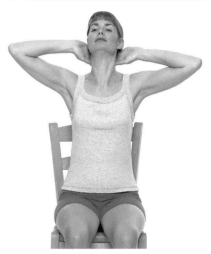

RESISTED EXTENSION
Sitting upright on a chair, bend your arms and place your fingers at the base of your skull, on either side of your spine. Push your head back against your hands, using gentle hand pressure to resist the movement, so that your head does not move. Hold for 2 to 3 seconds, return to the start position and repeat.

FORWARD LEAN

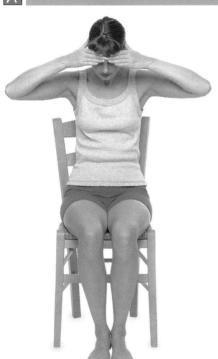

RESISTED FLEXION
Sitting upright on a chair, bend your arms and place your fingers on your forehead. Push your head forward against your hands, using gentle hand pressure to resist the movement. Hold, return to the start position and repeat.

NODDING

NECK STABILITY
Sit on the floor, with your back and "tail" against a wall and your legs stretched out in front of you. Gently bend your head down toward your chest, keeping the back of your head in contact with the wall and your chin level (not poking out, up or down). The movement should come from the back of your neck, at the top of your spine. Return to the start position and repeat.

INTERMEDIATE EXERCISES

Move on to these exercises only when you can do the beginners' section comfortably. Some are similar to those you have done already, but slightly more demanding. Aim for 6 to 8 repeats unless otherwise stated.

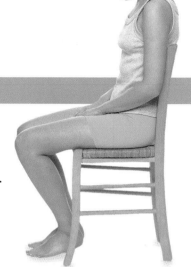

BACKWARD BEND

EXTENSION

Sit on a chair, with your shoulders and neck relaxed. Bend your head back, so that your chin points upward. Relax and repeat. Use one hand to support either side of your head if this is more comfortable.

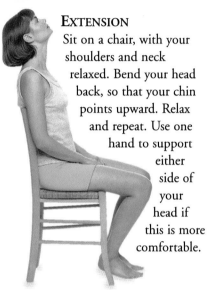

FORWARD BEND

FLEXION

Sit on a chair, with your shoulders and neck relaxed. Bend your head down toward your chest, tucking your chin in. Relax and repeat.

HEAD TILTS

SIDE FLEXION

1 Sit on a chair, with your shoulders and neck relaxed. Drop your head down to the left, bringing your left ear toward your left shoulder, as far as is comfortable. Return to the start position and repeat.
2 Repeat the same exercise, dropping your right ear down toward your right shoulder, as far as is comfortable.
The exercises on this page aim to enhance the mobility of the neck in all directions.

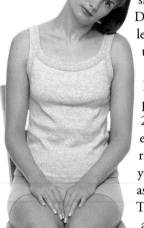

HEAD TURNS

ROTATION

Sit on a chair, with your shoulders and neck relaxed. Turn your head to the left, trying to look over your shoulder, as far as is comfortable. Return to the start position and repeat. Repeat the same exercise turning your head to the right to look over your right shoulder.

1

2

HEAD TILTS

LOCALIZED SIDE FLEXION

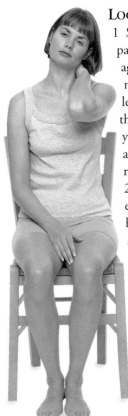

1 Sitting on a chair, place the palm of your left hand against the left side of your neck. Tilt your head to the left, keeping your hand in the same position. Keep your shoulders relaxed and down. Relax and repeat.

2 Repeat the same exercise using your right hand against the right side of your neck.

1

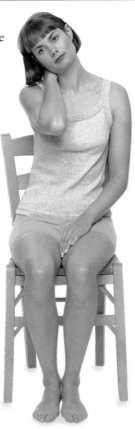

2

BACKWARD BEND

LOCALIZED EXTENSION

Sitting on a chair, link your hands behind your neck to support it. Tilt your head back over both hands. Relax and repeat.

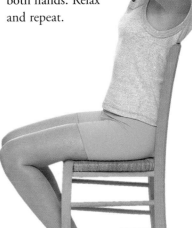

HEAD TURNS

LOCALIZED ROTATION

1 Sitting on a chair, place the palm of your left hand against the left side of your neck. Turn your head to the left, keeping your hand in the same position. Keep your shoulders relaxed. Relax and repeat.

2 Repeat the same exercise using your right hand against the right side of your neck.

The exercises on this page use the hand to localize movement in the spinal joints of the upper region of the neck, enabling you to concentrate on a specific area that is causing problems. For example, if your problem is on the left side, you may have more difficulty turning your head to the left.

1

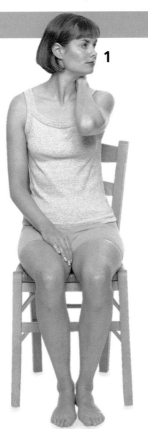

2

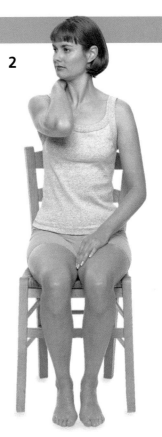

BACK PIVOT

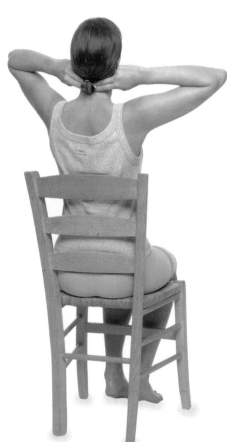

LOCALIZED EXTENSION

Sit on a chair with both hands behind your neck. Place your fingertips at the top of your neck, pointing in toward your spine and overlapping. Push up and in with your fingertips as you bring your head back. Return to vertical and repeat.

SIDE TWISTS

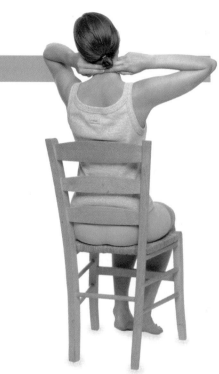

LOCALIZED EXTENSION WITH LATERAL FLEXION

Sit on a chair with hands behind your neck. Place your fingertips at the top of your neck, pointing in toward your spine and overlapping. Push up and in with your fingertips as you tilt your head to the left and back. Return to vertical, repeat, then repeat tilting your head to the right and back. This highlights an area of stiffness on one side of the neck. Variation: repeat the exercise tilting your head first to one side and then the other.

POSTURAL RETRAINING

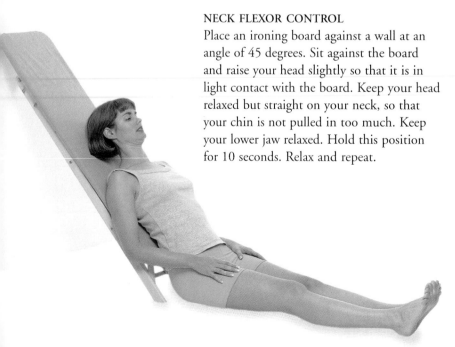

NECK FLEXOR CONTROL

Place an ironing board against a wall at an angle of 45 degrees. Sit against the board and raise your head slightly so that it is in light contact with the board. Keep your head relaxed but straight on your neck, so that your chin is not pulled in too much. Keep your lower jaw relaxed. Hold this position for 10 seconds. Relax and repeat.

BACKWARD STRETCH

LOCALIZED EXTENSION

Sit on a chair with both hands behind your neck. Place your fingertips at the top of your neck, pointing in toward your spine and overlapping. Gently draw your head and neck back against your fingers. Return to vertical and repeat.

NECK SCRUNCH

SEMISPINALIS CONTROL

1 Lie face down on the floor, propped up on your elbows, and drop your head down.

2 From this position, draw your head and neck up and back to straighten your spine. Push up through your shoulders and don't let your back sag. Keep your chin the same distance from your chest throughout the movement; holding a pair of rolled-up socks lightly under your chin will help you to do this. Hold the position, relax and repeat.

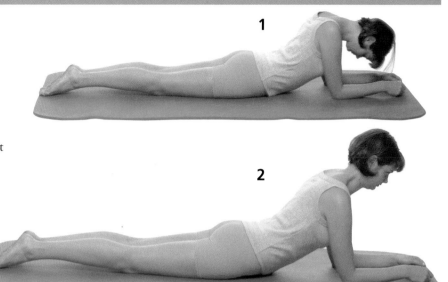

ASSISTED PIVOT

Sit on a chair holding a towel behind your neck. Use the towel as a pivot as you stretch your neck backward, so that you feel the movement in your neck vertebrae at the point where the towel presses against them. Return to the start position and repeat.

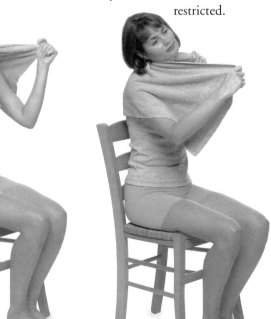

ASSISTED SIDE PIVOTS

Sit on a chair holding a towel behind your neck. Use the towel as a pivot to turn your neck to the left, return and repeat.

Repeat the exercise using the towel to turn your neck to the right.

Variation: do the exercise on both sides, concentrating on areas where you feel the movement is most restricted.

ASSISTED NECK TILTS

Sit on a chair holding a towel behind your neck. Use the towel to tilt your neck to the left. Return to the start position and repeat.

Repeat the exercise using the towel to tilt your neck to the right.

Variation: do the exercise on both sides, concentrating on areas where you feel the movement is most restricted.

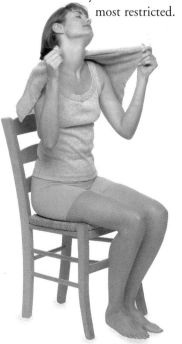

ADVANCED EXERCISES

Move on to these exercises when you are comfortable with the intermediate ones. You should be able to achieve almost the full range of movement in your neck and tolerate a greater stretch than before. Repeat the strengthening exercises until fatigued.

BACKWARD BEND

EXTENSION

Sit on a chair and lean your head back to its comfortable limit. Keep your shoulders relaxed. Do not hold the position. Bring your head gently and smoothly back to vertical. Repeat up to 4 times.

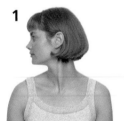

FORWARD BEND

FLEXION

Sit on a chair and nod your head down to your chest. Don't poke or tuck your chin in – keep it in the same position throughout the movement. Bring your head gently back to a vertical position and repeat up to 4 times.

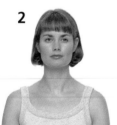

HEAD TILTS

SIDE FLEXION

Sit on a chair and, keeping your head facing forward, tilt your head to your left shoulder as far as is comfortable. Return to the upright position and repeat.

Then repeat the sequence, tilting your head to your right shoulder as far as is comfortable. Variation: do the exercise on alternate sides. You may like to do this exercise in front of a mirror so that you can watch the movement as you do it and ensure that you do not lean forward or back.

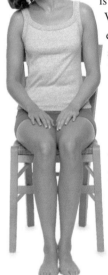

HEAD TURNS

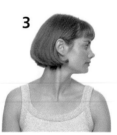

1   **2**   **3**

ROTATIONS

1 Sit on a chair and turn your head to the right as far as is comfortable.
2 Return to face forward and repeat.
3 Repeat the same exercise turning your head to the left as far as is comfortable. Repeat the sequence up to 5 times.
Variation: Do the exercise on both sides, concentrating on areas where you feel the movement is most restricted.

FORWARD BEND

FLEXION

Sit on the floor with your legs straight out in front of you and your back straight. Slump forward, bending your neck so that your chin comes down toward your chest. Relax and repeat 3 to 4 times.

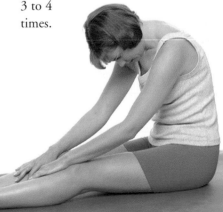
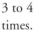

BACKWARD BEND

EXTENSION

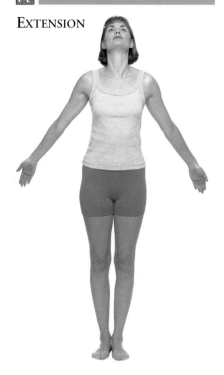

Stand straight with your arms extended. Keeping your arms in this position, take your head back, bending your neck to a comfortable limit. Relax and repeat 5 times.

BACKWARD STRETCH

ANTERIOR FLEXIBILITY

1 Sit in front of a mirror with the arm on your weak side hanging down toward the floor, palm facing in and hand relaxed but open.
2 Keeping your shoulder and neck relaxed, move your arm slightly behind you and raise it to an angle of about 70 degrees from your body. Keep your neck in a "neutral" position, not tilted to one side or the other. Hold, relax and repeat up to 3 times.

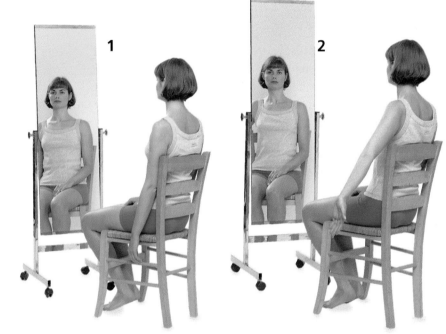

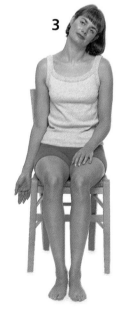

HEAD TILTS

MUSCLE RELAXATION

1 Sit on a chair with the hand on your weak side pointing to the floor, palm turned outward. Tilt your head to the other side.
2 Push your arm toward the floor and lift your strong shoulder as you take a deep breath in.
3 Hold the breath for 5 seconds. Breathe out and let your arm relax. The stretch in your neck should have increased, allowing your arm to drop further. Repeat up to 4 times. Variation: Do the exercise on both sides, concentrating on areas where the movement is most restricted.

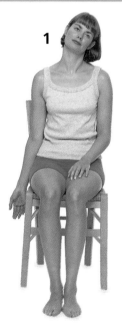

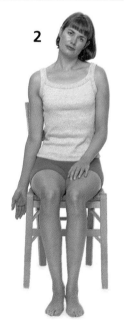

NECK BENDS

NECK FLEXION

1 Lie on your back with your head on a folded towel.
2 Lift your head off the floor, keeping your chin
tucked in to your chest. Hold for 1 to 2 seconds
and then bend your neck to its comfortable limit for a
further 1 to 2 seconds, still keeping your chin tucked in.
Gently uncurl your neck, lowering your head to the floor.
As your neck becomes stronger, hold for up to 5 seconds;
you can also hold the position at as many different points
through the range as are comfortable.

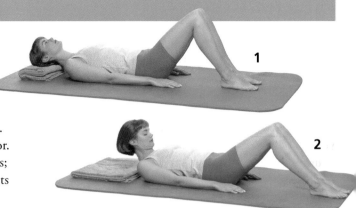

 ## HEAD RAISES

SIDE FLEXION

1 Lie on your side with your head resting on a
folded towel.
2 Lift your head up slightly, without moving it
forward or back. Hold for 1–2 seconds and then lift
your head as high as is comfortable for a further 1 to 2
seconds. Gently lower your head. As your neck becomes
stronger, maintain the holds for up to 5 seconds; you can
also hold the position at as many different points
through the range as is comfortable.
Repeat the same exercise lying on your other side.

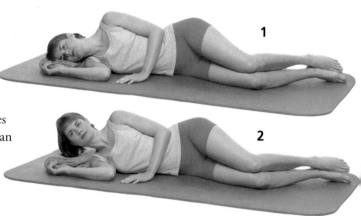

HEAD RAISES

RETRACTION

1 Sit on a chair, with your feet flat on the floor.
2 Lean back in the chair, keeping your head straight on
your neck. Do not force this – go back only as far as is
comfortable. Don't poke your chin out or tuck it in.
Hold the position for 1 to 2 seconds, relax and repeat.

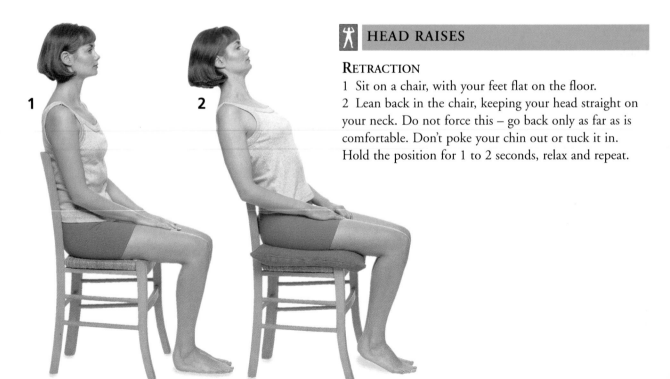

LOWER NECK STRETCH

SEMISPINALIS

1 Stand with hands and forearms resting on a table. Lean forward with your neck and back slightly bent.
2 Keeping your chin in, draw your head and neck back, straightening your spine; feel the muscles between your shoulders and in your lower neck working. Hold for 1 to 2 seconds, relax and repeat. It may feel awkward – the key is to move your head without letting your chin poke.

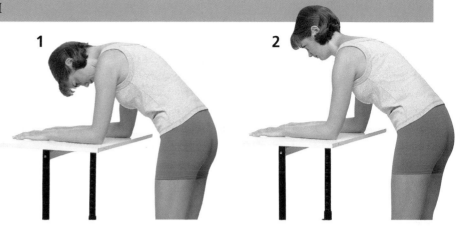

LOWER NECK SRETCH

NECK EXTENSION

1 Start on your hands and knees, with your shoulders directly over your hands. Drop your head down. Hold.
2 Raise your head so that your back is straight from head to "tail". Hold. Repeat the exercise a few times.

Variation: place a thin book on your head to help you to keep your neck straight in the upper position.

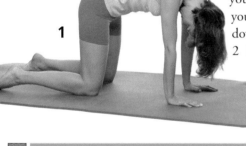
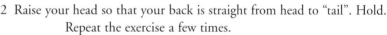

TWIST UPS

FLEXION WITH ROTATION

1 Lie on your back with your head on a folded towel. Without raising your shoulders off the ground, lift your head up and turn it to the right. Hold for 1 to 2 seconds, return your head to the centre, then lift it as high as is comfortable and turn to the right for a further 1 to 2 seconds. Return to the centre and gently lower your head to the floor. As your neck becomes stronger, maintain the holds for up to 5 seconds; you can also hold the position at as many different points as are comfortable.
2 Variation: repeat the sequence turning your neck to the left.

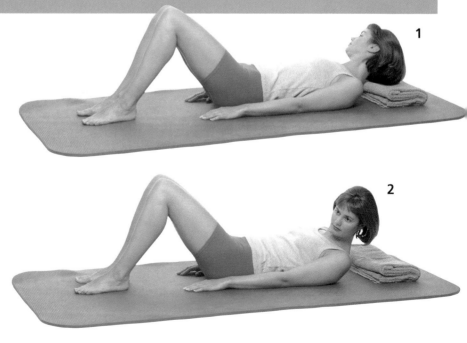

Upper Back Exercises

Like all regions of the spine, the upper back consists of a series of interlocking blocks (vertebrae), each linked on either side by a facet joint. Each vertebra also has a disc connecting the body of one vertebra to the next. With so many different elements, there are many places where things can go wrong. Just as one or more discs may cause pain, a single facet joint may be stiff, on one or both sides, or several may be involved. So pain may be confined to a small area, or it may restrict a number of different movements. With upper back problems, you will usually feel pain in a specific area and have trouble with a particular movement – turning to put on your seat belt, for example. It can be difficult to tell which exercises are best for your spine problem. Particularly if the pain is severe, start very gently, and consult a professional if you are in any doubt that you are doing the right thing.

HOW TO GET STARTED

• Start with the beginners' exercises for mobility. If you can do them all easily, try the beginners' exercises for flexibility, then those for strength and stability. If they are all easy, move on to the intermediate level.

• If at any stage you find an exercise is difficult – either because it hurts or because you cannot do the movement – you have identified a problem area. Work through the rest of the exercises at that level and see if any more are difficult. Repeat those particular exercises every day and you should find they become easier.

• Work on one level of exercises only. Do not attempt any at the intermediate level until you can do all the beginners' exercises comfortably. The same applies when you progress from the intermediate to the advanced level.

BEGINNERS' EXERCISES

These exercises aim to introduce early mobility into the upper back, while encouraging muscle control of the movements and ensuring adequate flexibility in the soft tissues. Do not do any of these exercises to the point of pain, and do not force yourself to do anything that is not comfortable. Work gradually and steadily through the exercises – there is no benefit to be gained from pushing your body to do things for which it is not ready.

UPPER BACK STRETCHES & TURNS

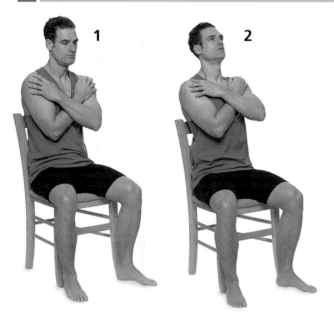

Throughout this sequence, movement should come from the middle and upper part of your back. At the comfortable limit of each movement, hold gently.

Sit on a chair with your arms crossed on your chest and your hands on your shoulders (1). Keeping your chin tucked in, bend gently forward, then back (2). Tilt to the right side (3), then to the left (4); turn your upper body to the right (5), then to the left (6). Repeat the sequence.

This exercise increases mobility in all directions in this section of the spine.

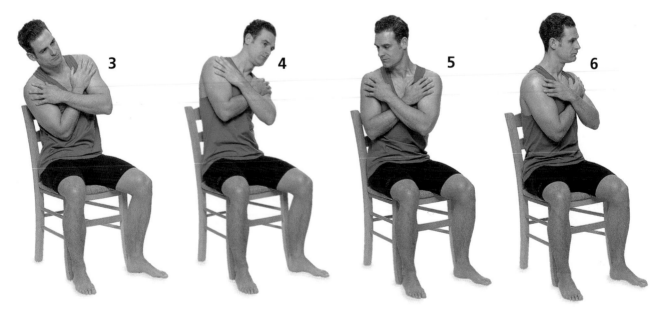

THE CAT

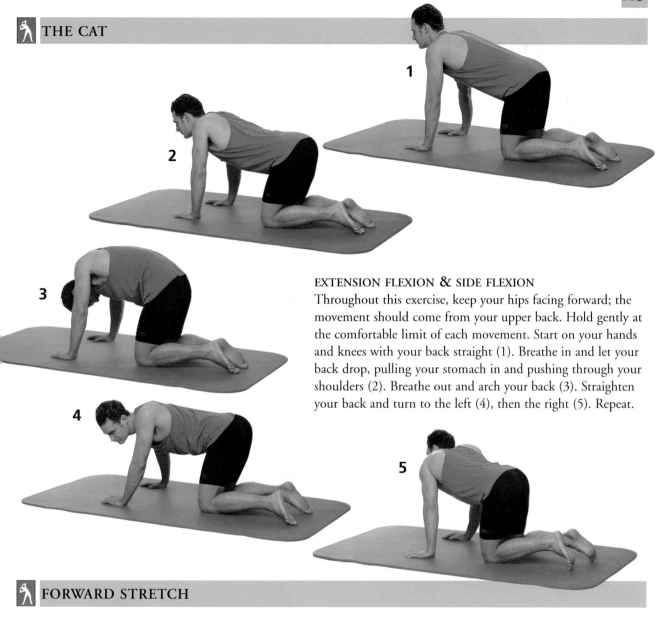

EXTENSION FLEXION & SIDE FLEXION

Throughout this exercise, keep your hips facing forward; the movement should come from your upper back. Hold gently at the comfortable limit of each movement. Start on your hands and knees with your back straight (1). Breathe in and let your back drop, pulling your stomach in and pushing through your shoulders (2). Breathe out and arch your back (3). Straighten your back and turn to the left (4), then the right (5). Repeat.

FORWARD STRETCH

FLEXION/EXTENSION

1 Kneel on the floor, sitting back on your heels.
2 Bend forward from your hips to put your hands on the floor with your arms straight, then alternately "round" and "flatten" your back. Repeat as often as is comfortable.

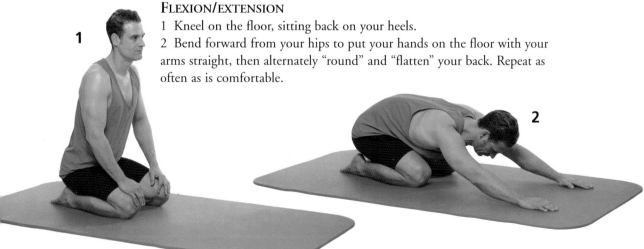

BACKWARD BEND

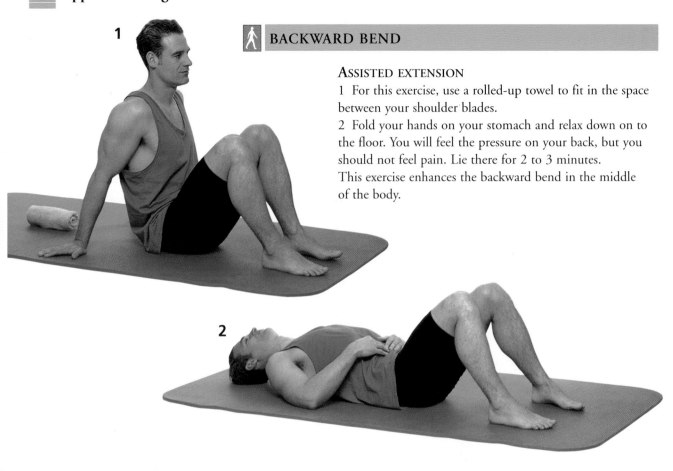

ASSISTED EXTENSION

1 For this exercise, use a rolled-up towel to fit in the space between your shoulder blades.

2 Fold your hands on your stomach and relax down on to the floor. You will feel the pressure on your back, but you should not feel pain. Lie there for 2 to 3 minutes.

This exercise enhances the backward bend in the middle of the body.

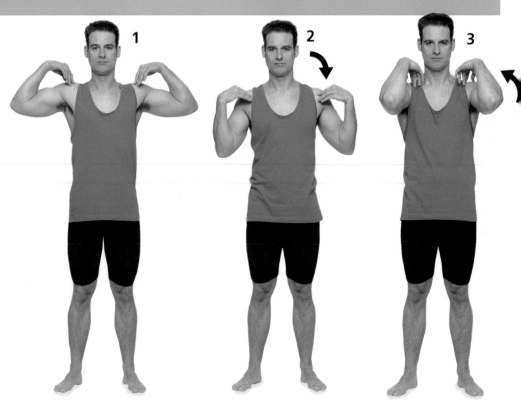

ARM CIRCLES

1 Stand with your elbows bent and hands on your shoulders.

2 Circle both arms forward.

3 Then reverse the movement and circle both arms back.

Repeat up to 20 times, working the muscles around the shoulder blades and upper back.

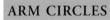

ARM EXTENSIONS

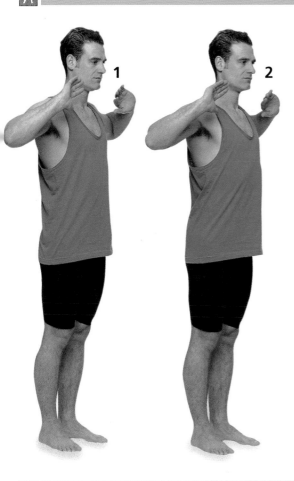

SCAPULAR RETRACTION

1 Stand with your arms bent, in line with your shoulders, and your palms facing forward.

2 Take your elbows back as far as is comfortable so that you feel a squeeze between your shoulder blades. Gently hold and repeat.

NECK STABILITY

Place an ironing board at a 60-degree angle to the wall. Sit on the floor so that your shoulder blades are flat against the board and the back of your skull is lightly touching it. Try to maintain the position without letting your lower back flatten against the board. Hold the position for a count of between 10 and 60 seconds. Feel the muscles in your neck and upper back working to maintain this posture.

SUPPORTED HEAD RAISES

SEMISPINALIS CONTROL

1 Lean your forearms on a table with your head hanging down and your neck relaxed.

2 Gently draw your head back and up, keeping your chin tucked in. The effort should come from between your upper back and shoulders.

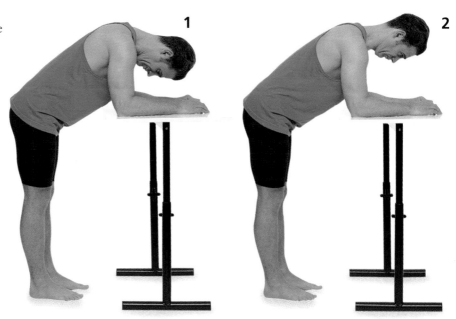

INTERMEDIATE EXERCISES

Move on to these exercises when you can do the beginners' ones without discomfort. Your upper back should be stronger and more flexible, and you should be able to hold positions for longer than a few seconds. Unless otherwise stated, aim for 6 to 8 repeats of each exercise.

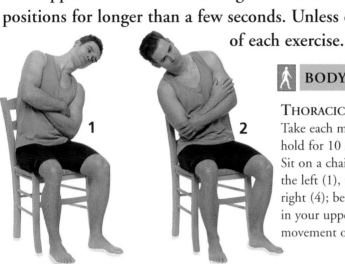

BODY STRETCH

THORACIC MOBILITY

Take each movement in this exercise to its comfortable limit and hold for 10 seconds.

Sit on a chair, with your arms folded on your stomach. Bend to the left (1), then to the right (2); turn to the left (3), then to the right (4); bend backward (5), then forward (6), feeling the stretch in your upper back. Repeat the sequence, or any individual movement on which you feel you need to concentrate.

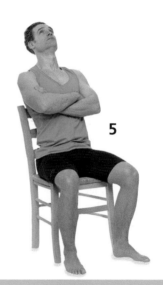

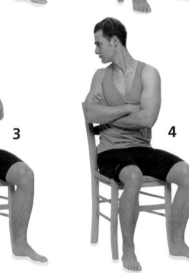

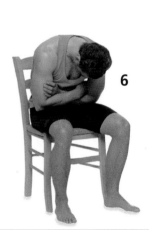

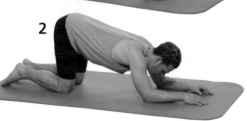

FOUR-POINT KNEEL

WEIGHT-BEARING THORACIC EXTENSION

Take each movement in this exercise to its comfortable limit.

1 Start on your hands and knees, with your knees in line with your hips.

2 Lean forward to rest on your forearms so that your back is straight.

3 Sit back toward your heels, straightening your arms out in front of you to stretch your upper back. Keep your chin tucked in. Hold and repeat the sequence.

ASSISTED BENDS

LOCALIZED EXTENSION, ROTATION & LATERAL FLEXIBILITY

This movement comes from your upper back; take each stage to its comfortable limit and hold. Sitting on a chair, hold a bath towel by its top corners so that it is taut behind you. Use it as a pivot as you bend backward (**1**), then rotate (**2**) and bend (**3**) to left and right. Repeat the sequence, or any part you feel is appropriate.

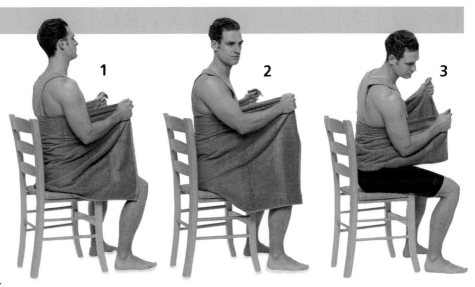

BACK STRETCH

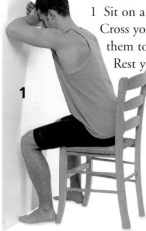

ASSISTED EXTENSION

1 Sit on a chair facing a wall. Cross your arms and lift them to lean on the wall. Rest your head on your forearms.

2 Breathe in and feel your back curl away from the wall. Then relax and breathe out, to let your upper back drop down and extend. Repeat up to 5 times.

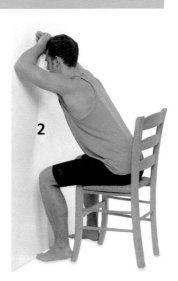

SIDE STRETCH

Stand sideways on to a doorway with one arm slightly elevated and the forearm resting on the frame. Press your forearm into the frame. Twist your trunk away from the frame, leaving your arm in the same position. Keep your shoulder down and relaxed. Rest and repeat, then repeat the sequence with the other arm.

SIDE STRETCHES

1 Stand with your back to a wall, arms crossed above your head and in contact with the wall.

2 & 3 Slowly bend from side to side, keeping your arms in contact with the wall. Feel the stretch in your sides as you bend. Make sure that you keep your lower back steady – don't let it "give".

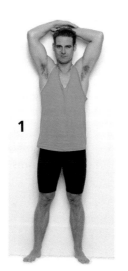
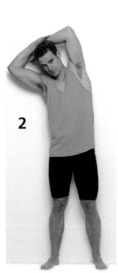
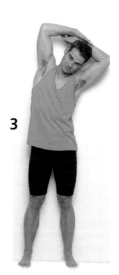

UPWARD LIFT

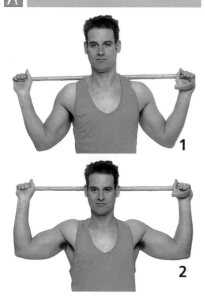

ASSISTED ELEVATION

1 Stand with a broom or a walking stick across the back of your shoulders.

2 Lift the stick up to ear level, without poking your chin out, and keep your shoulders relaxed. Keep your lower back steady as you lift – don't let it "give". Try the exercise sitting on a chair if you find it easier.

UPWARD SLIDE

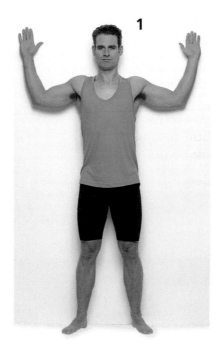
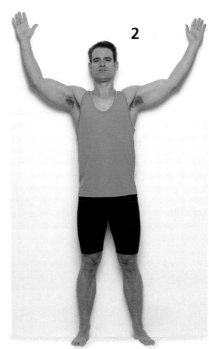

SCAPULAR CONTROL

1 Stand with your back to a wall. Bring your arms out to the side, slightly raised, with your elbows bent and your arms touching the wall.

2 Slowly slide your arms up the wall, keeping your arms and shoulder blades in contact with it. Keep your lower back steady and your stomach pulled up and in.

PUSH-UPS

BALANCE

On your hands and knees, lean forward and backward on your arms, keeping your lower back steady by pulling your stomach up and in. You may feel a stretch in your arms as you lean forward and in your thighs as you lean back, but you should not feel any strain in the back itself. Keep the movements small so that you do not wobble: at the start position your hands should be beneath your shoulders. Repeat until fatigued.

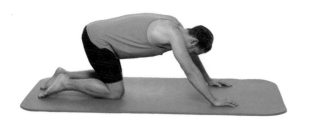

SHOULDER LIFT

LOWER TRAPEZIUS

Lie on your front, with your arms by your side and your head straight and supported by a rolled-up towel. In one smooth movement, lift first your hands, then your elbows and finally your shoulders, so that your arms are still straight by your sides, but raised about 20 cm (8 in) off the floor. Hold for 10 seconds and repeat. Remember to keep your shoulders off the floor; as you get tired they will tend to drop. Aim for 10 repetitions of a 10-second hold, although it may be easier to start with 10 repetitions of a 2-second hold and build up to 10 seconds.

WEIGHT TRANSFERENCE

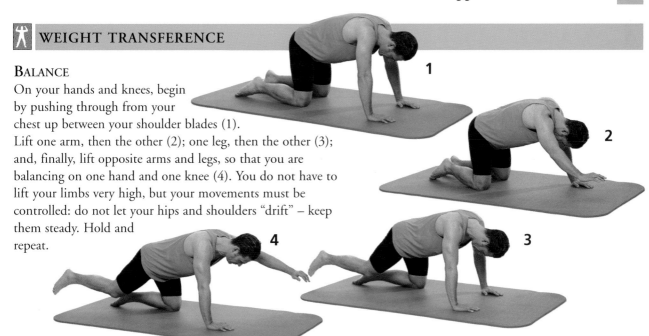

BALANCE

On your hands and knees, begin by pushing through from your chest up between your shoulder blades (1).
Lift one arm, then the other (2); one leg, then the other (3); and, finally, lift opposite arms and legs, so that you are balancing on one hand and one knee (4). You do not have to lift your limbs very high, but your movements must be controlled: do not let your hips and shoulders "drift" – keep them steady. Hold and repeat.

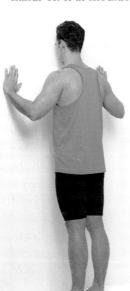

BODY LIFT

FOUR-POINT PRESS-UPS

On your hands and knees, lower and raise your body by bending and straightening your elbows. Repeat until fatigued, working the muscles in the shoulder blades and upper back.

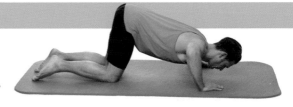

SHOULDER CLENCH

SCAPULAR CONTROL

Stand facing a wall, with both arms raised, the sides of your hands against the wall and your thumbs pointing away from it. Pull your shoulder blades down and back. Hold, relax and repeat.

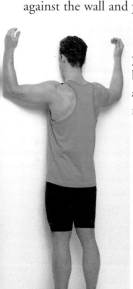

VERTICAL PRESS-UPS

SCAPULAR CONTROL

Stand facing a wall, with your feet slightly away from it, and your hands on it at shoulder level. Keeping your feet still, bend and stretch your arms. Repeat until fatigued.

SHOULDER SQUEEZE

SCAPULAR CONTROL

Stand with your back to a wall, your elbows bent at 90 degrees and your upper arms against the wall. Push away from the wall by squeezing your shoulder blades together and pushing through with your upper back. These three exercises work the muscles which stabilize the shoulder blades and upper back.

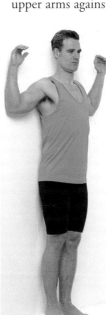

ADVANCED EXERCISES

By the time you move on to these exercises, you should be able to do all the intermediate exercises comfortably and achieve almost the full range of movement in your upper back. Repeat the strengthening exercises until fatigued.

 ## BODY TWISTS & BENDS

ROTATION & SIDE FLEXION

1 Sit on a chair. Put one arm across your body to hold the back of the chair on the opposite side. Pull against the chair as you turn your body toward the hand holding the chair. Hold and repeat on both sides.
2 Keeping your shoulders square, bend to the left, letting your left arm hang down. Hold and repeat the exercise on both sides.

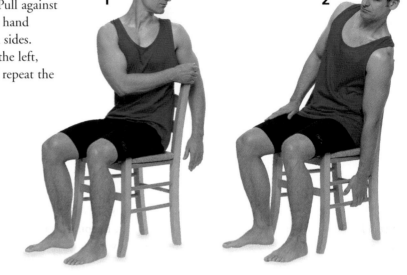

UPWARD STRETCH

EXTENSION

Sit on a chair with your arms raised above your head, palms facing up and fingers linked. Stretch your arms out behind you as you lean over the back of the chair. Hold and repeat.

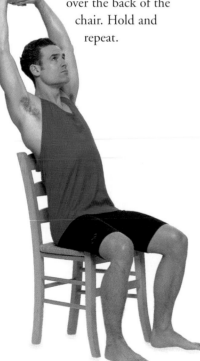

BODY TWIST

ASSISTED ROTATION

Sit on a chair and turn your upper body to the right, using your right arm to help you turn by gently swinging it out to the side and up. Then turn your upper body to the left, using your left arm in the same way. Repeat.

SIDEWAYS BENDS

LATERAL FLEXION

Stand with your arms
linked behind you
with your palms facing
inward and lean first to
the left, then to the right,
keeping your body in line.
Take the position as far as is
comfortable on each side.
Repeat.

This exercise increases
mobility in the upper
back and between the
shoulder blades.

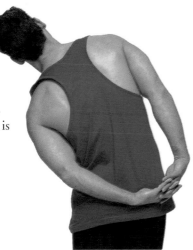

BACKWARD STRETCH

RETRACTION & EXTENSION

Stand with arms linked behind
you, palms facing inward. Look
up as you stretch your arms
behind you. Keep your stomach
up and in and don't let your
chin poke out as you squeeze
your shoulder blades together.
Repeat with palms facing
outward.

Like the previous exercise, this
increases mobility in the upper
back and between the shoulder
blades.

SALUTE TO THE SUN

THROUGH RANGE FLEXION & EXTENSION

Do this exercise as one continuous movement to improve mobility and
flexibility through your upper back.

On your hands and knees, shift your weight forward, bending your arms (1).
Straighten your arms as you straighten your whole body, lifting your chest up
(2). This should be a smooth "swooping" movement. Keeping your hands in
the same position, bend your knees and hips so that you finish in a kneel-
sitting position (3). Repeat.

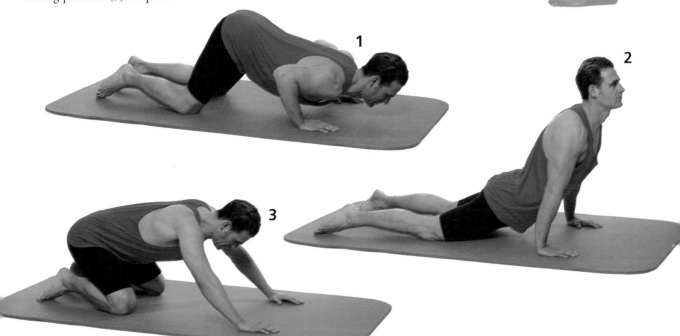

BODY STRETCH

THORACIC EXTENSION

Lie on your back with your legs bent and your arms on the floor above your head, close to your ears. Keep your back flat and if your arms don't touch the floor, use a rolled-up towel under each arm to support it in a comfortable extended position. Relax into the position for 1 to 3 minutes.

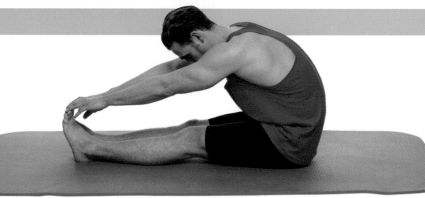

 ## LONG-SITTING SLUMP

Sit on the floor with your legs straight out in front of you. Slump forward, keeping your arms straight and your chin tucked in. Hold and repeat. Don't worry if you can't touch your toes. Feel the stretch through the length of your spine and into your legs.

FORWARD STRETCH

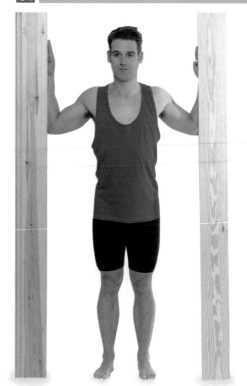

ASSISTED THORACIC EXTENSION

Stand in a doorway with both arms raised and resting against the door frame. Your elbows should be at an angle of about 90 degrees and your hands level with your head. Press your hands against the door frame as you lean your upper body through the doorway. Feel a stretch through the front of your shoulders and upper back as you reach the limit of the movement. Hold, relax and repeat.

BACKWARD STRETCH

ANTERIOR FLEXIBILITY

Stand with one arm extended and slightly out to the side. Keep your head and neck straight and make sure your shoulder does not lift up as you raise your arm to a comfortable limit behind you. The movement should come from your shoulder blade. Hold, relax and repeat, alternating arms, until fatigued.

LEG LIFT

1 Lie on whichever side is more comfortable with your elbow bent and head supported on your hand. Place your other hand in on the floor in front of your chest to support you.

2 Breathe out as you lift both legs off the floor. Keep them straight and in line with your body. Hold, relax and repeat a few times, then turn over and repeat on the other side. You should feel the muscles in your waist working.

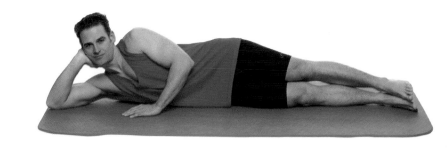

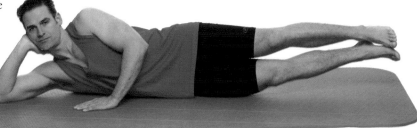

 TWO-POINT BALANCE

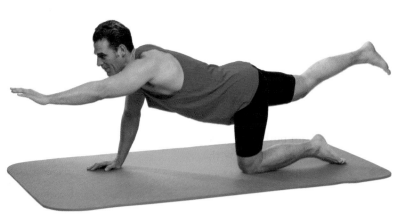

On your hands and knees, pull your stomach up and in, then lift opposite arms and legs and stretch them out in front and behind you so that you are balancing on one hand and the opposite knee. Keep your back straight and steady, and lift your limbs to keep them in line with your back. Hold, relax and repeat with the other hand and knee.

PRESS-UPS

Lie on your front with your toes tucked under, your hands under your shoulders and your elbows bent. Straighten your arms to lift your body off the floor, keeping your back, hips and legs straight. Repeat by bending and straightening your arms until fatigued. You should feel the muscles working in your arms and upper back.

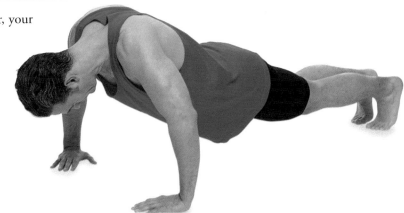

ARM LIFT

UPPER THORACIC STABILITY

1 Lie on your front with your head to one side, arms slightly bent and shoulder blades pulled down and back.

2 Lift your arms off the floor and hold for 3 to 5 seconds. Relax and repeat.

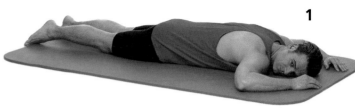

1

2

 BACK STRETCH

SPINAL EXTENSORS

Lie on your front with your head to one side. Your arms should be straight, with your thumbs pointing up and your shoulder blades pulled down and back. Either bend your knees or keep your legs flat on the floor. Lift your arms off the floor, keeping them as straight as possible, and hold for 3 to 5 seconds. Keep your head down. Relax and repeat.

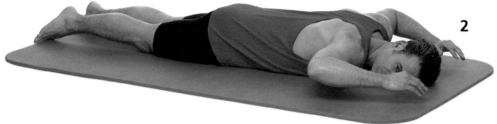

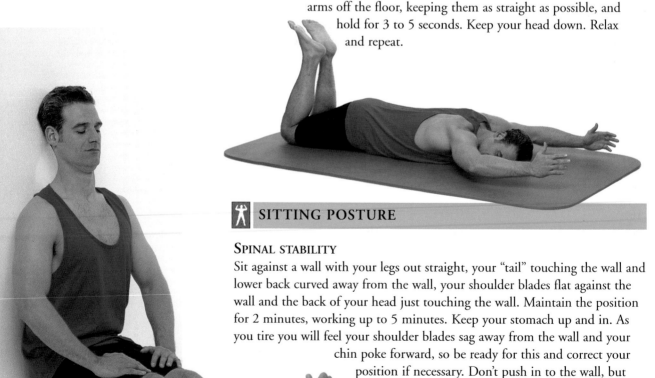

SITTING POSTURE

SPINAL STABILITY

Sit against a wall with your legs out straight, your "tail" touching the wall and lower back curved away from the wall, your shoulder blades flat against the wall and the back of your head just touching the wall. Maintain the position for 2 minutes, working up to 5 minutes. Keep your stomach up and in. As you tire you will feel your shoulder blades sag away from the wall and your chin poke forward, so be ready for this and correct your position if necessary. Don't push in to the wall, but use it to remind you of the aim of the exercise – to strengthen your postural muscles – and to help you correct your position.

SHOULDER CONTROL

THORACIC & SCAPULAR CONTROL

Wearing or holding small wrist weights, stand with your arms straight out to the side. Use small repetitive movements upward (1), backward and to circle your arms forward and then backward (2). Keep your stomach up and in and don't let your chin poke out.

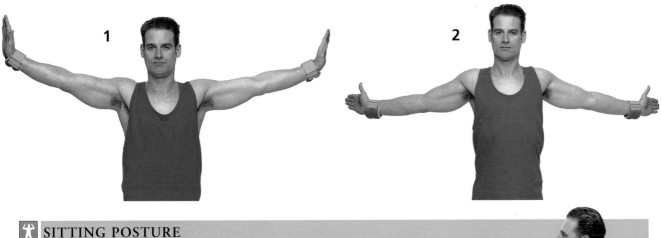

SITTING POSTURE

LONG SITTING STABILITY

Sit up straight with your legs straight out in front of you. Maintain the position for 2 minutes, working up to 5 minutes. Keep your stomach pulled up and in. As you tire you will feel your shoulder blades sag and your chin poke forward, so be ready for this and correct your position if necessary.

SIT-UPS

ABDOMINALS

Lie on your back in a relaxed position. As you breathe out, bring your head up to look down your body, raising your chest and arms slightly off the floor. Keep your feet relaxed. Hold, relax and repeat. This strengthens the abdominal muscles which support the back.

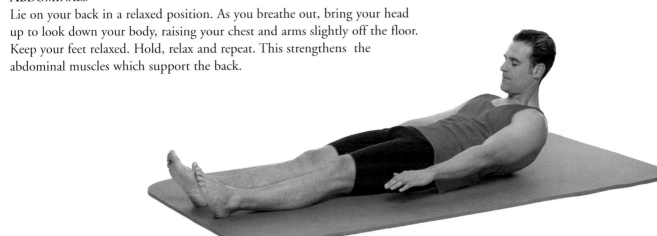

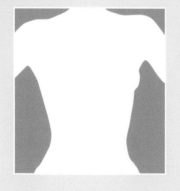

Lower Back Exercises

The basic structure of the spine, explained on page 112, can cause similar problems in the lower back. Again, the pain may be localised or widespread, with different movements feeling restricted. You may feel pain in one side of your lower back when you bend to put on your shoes, for example, or in the middle after you have been standing for prolonged periods of time. The exercises in this chapter are designed to cover a number of different types of problem, taking you through a routine that will restore the maximum range of movement in your lower back, as well as flexibility in the soft tissues and strength in the supporting muscles. It can sometimes be difficult to tell which exercises are best for an individual complaint. Particularly if the pain is severe, work very cautiously and progress gently. Consult a professional if you are in any doubt that you are doing the right thing.

HOW TO GET STARTED

• Start with the beginners' exercises for mobility. If you can do them all easily, try the beginners' exercises for flexibility, then those for strength and stability. If they are all easy, move on to the intermediate level.

• If at any stage you find an exercise is difficult – either because it hurts or because you cannot do the movement – you have identified a problem area. Work through the rest of the exercises at that level and see if any more are difficult. Repeat those particular exercises every day and you should find they become easier.

• Work on one level of exercises only. Do not attempt any at the intermediate level until you can do all the beginners' exercises comfortably. The same applies when you progress from the intermediate to the advanced level.

MOBILITY

BEGINNER
Leg bends	130
Hip rolls	130
Pelvic tilt	130
Push-ups	131
Sideways stretches	131
Sideways bend	132

INTERMEDIATE
Side glide	134
Push-ups	134
Forward drop	134
Side drops	135

ADVANCED
Full back stretch	138
Spinal mobility	138

FLEXIBILITY

BEGINNER
Upward push	131
Sideways pushes	131
Wall push-ups	132
Pelvic tilt	133

INTERMEDIATE
Hip rolls	134
Forward lean	135
Body curl	135
Pelvic stretch	135
"The waiter's bow"	136

ADVANCED
Thigh stretch	138
Forward stretch	139
Advanced slump	139
Thigh stretch	139

STRENGTH & STABILITY

BEGINNER
Bent knee drop	132
Heel slide	133
Tummy tuck	133
Heel squeeze	133

INTERMEDIATE
Forward slump	136
Knee bends	136
Bent knee lift	136
Muscle tone	137
Supine cycling	137
Leg straightening	137

ADVANCED
Side scrunch	139
Double leg lift	140
Backward leg lift	140
Double leg twists	140
Muscle tightening	140
Advanced leg lift	140
Curl downs	141
Straight leg lift	141
Twist sit-ups	141

BEGINNERS' EXERCISES

These exercises are your first steps toward strengthening your lower back and restoring its flexibility and mobility. Repeat each exercise only as often as is comfortable – if something hurts, you may need to go more gently.

 LEG BENDS

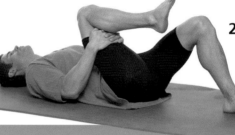

ASSISTED LUMBAR FLEXION

1 Lie on your back with one leg bent at the knee and foot flat on the floor. Clasp your hands under your other thigh, bend the knee and lift the leg.
2 Use your hands to help you pull the knee as close to your chest as is comfortable. Reverse legs and do the exercise again. Repeat a few times, as often as is comfortable.

HIP ROLLS

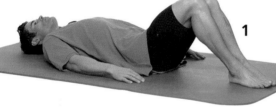

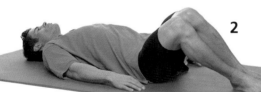

LUMBAR ROTATION

1 Lie on your back with your knees bent, feet and hands flat on the floor.
2 Keeping your knees together, let them drop down toward the floor, first to one side, then the other. Your feet should remain in contact with the floor. Let each buttock in turn rise slightly off the floor as you roll from side to side. Repeat a few times, as often as is comfortable.

PELVIC TILT

LUMBAR FLEXION & EXTENSION

1 Lie on your back, knees bent and feet together and flat on the floor.
2 Squeeze your buttocks and feel your lower back arch off the floor. Hold for 1 to 2 seconds, then relax. Try to make the movement smooth and take it as far as is comfortable. Repeat a few times, then flatten your back on to the floor.

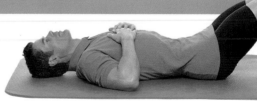

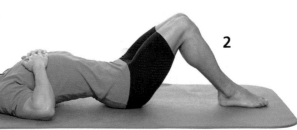

PUSH-UPS

LUMBAR EXTENSION

1 Lie on your front with your arms bent, hands about level with your nose, your legs straight and your toes on the floor.
2 Keeping your forearms on the floor, gently raise your upper arms so that you push your body up and arch your back. Keep your legs and back relaxed. Repeat as often as is comfortable.

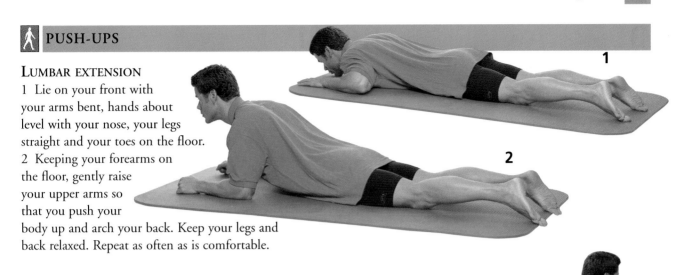

 SIDEWAYS STRETCHES

LATERAL EXTENSION

1 Start in the same position as above. Keeping your knees straight and together, slide both legs slightly to the right, then push up on your elbows.
2 Then slide your legs slightly to the left and push up on your elbows. Repeat a few times, as often as is comfortable.
Note Depending on the nature of your injury, you may be advised to do this exercise to one side only. Check with your physiotherapist or doctor.

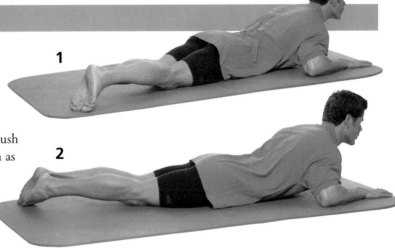

UPWARD PUSH

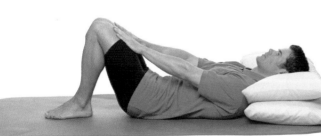

RESISTED ABDOMINALS

Lie on your back (with a couple of pillows under your head if this is more comfortable), with your hips and knees bent, and feet and knees slightly apart. Put your hands on your knees and, without moving your feet, try to push your knees against your hands. You should feel your stomach muscles working. Hold for a few seconds, relax and repeat.

SIDEWAYS PUSHES

RESISTED ABDOMINALS

Start in the same position as for the Upward Push, left. Put your right hand on the outside of your right knee and push against your hand with your knee. Hold, relax, repeat. Repeat with the left hand on the left side. The push should come from your stomach and you should feel a gentle stretch in your lower back.
Note Your physiotherapist may advise you to do this exercise to one side only.

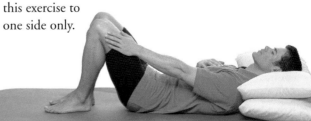

SIDEWAYS BEND

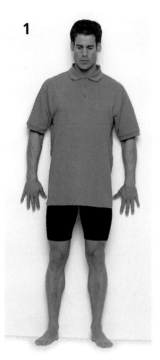

1

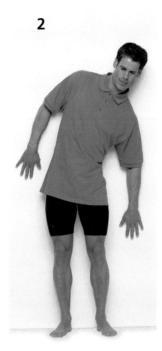

2

LATERAL FLEXION

1 Stand with your back to a wall.

2 Keeping your shoulders in contact with the wall and your back relaxed, lean down to one side. Straighten and repeat, then repeat to the other side.

Note You may be advised to do this exercise to one side only. Check with your physiotherapist or doctor.

WALL PUSH-UPS

EXTENSIONS

1 Stand facing a wall with your feet apart and slightly away from the wall, your hands flat on the wall and elbows bent.

2 Gently straighten your arms to push your upper body away from the wall so that your lower back arches. Hold for a few seconds, relax and repeat as often as is comfortable.

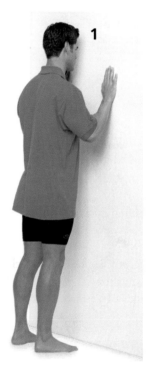

1

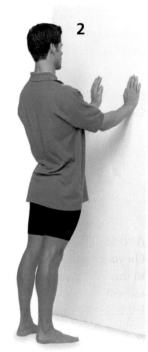

2

BENT KNEE DROP

TRUNK STABILITY

1 Lie on your back (with a pillow under your head if this is more comfortable), knees bent and your feet flat on the floor. Pull your stomach up and under your rib cage and draw your tummy button toward your spine.

2 Place your hands on the front of your pelvis, and gently let one leg roll out to the side, without your back "giving". Repeat a few times.

Note You may be advised to do this exercise to one side only. Check with your physiotherapist or doctor.

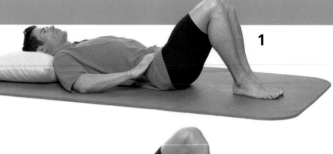

1

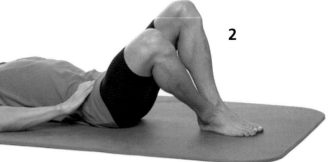

2

HEEL SLIDE

ABDOMINALS

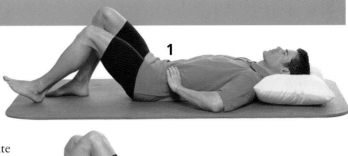

1 Lie on your back (with a pillow under your head if this is more comfortable), your knees bent and your feet flat on the floor. Pull your stomach up and under your ribcage, drawing your tummy button in toward your spine. Gently slide one heel a little way away from your body and bring it back again. Alternate with your left and right leg. Don't let your back "give".
2 Once you can do this 10 times without your back "giving", try lifting one foot at a time a little way off the floor, then both feet. Repeat as often as is comfortable.

TUMMY TUCK

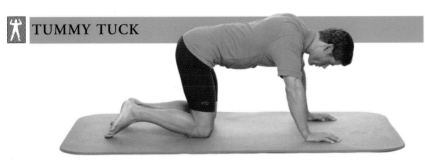

ABDOMINALS

On your hands and knees, pull your abdominal muscles up and in so that your tummy button moves toward your spine. Hold for a few seconds, relax, repeat. Remember to keep your back straight – don't let it sag when you relax.

HEEL SQUEEZE

ABDOMINALS

1 Lie on your front, with your knees bent and slightly apart, but your feet together.
2 Squeeze your heels together, so that your buttock muscles contract. Hold for 5 seconds, then relax and repeat. Keep the rest of your body relaxed.

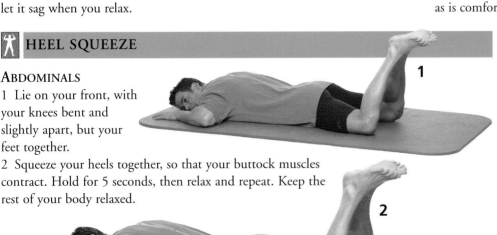

PELVIC TILT

LUMBAR FLEXIONS & EXTENSIONS
Stand with your back to a wall. Holding your hands on your stomach so that you can feel the movement, flatten your lower back against the wall and relax. Repeat as often as is comfortable.

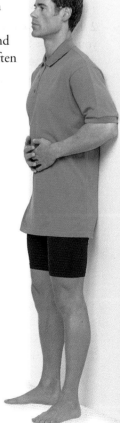

INTERMEDIATE EXERCISES

Do not attempt these exercises until you can do the beginners' ones easily and without discomfort. These exercises require greater mobility and muscle strength, and will produce a greater stretch in your lower back.

HIP ROLLS

ROTATION

1 Lie on your back with your knees bent, feet flat on the floor and hands on your stomach.
2 Keeping your knees together, let them drop toward the floor to one side. Lift your clasped hands to the other side, to increase the stretch. Your feet should remain in contact with the floor. Reverse the movement, dropping your knees and twisting your arms to the other side. Your buttocks should be raised slightly off the floor as you roll from side to side. Repeat a few times, as often as is comfortable.

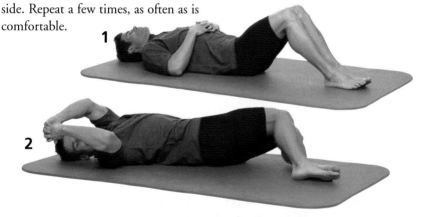

PUSH-UPS

EXTENSION

1 Lie on your front with arms bent, hands about level with your nose, your legs straight and your toes on the floor.
2 Gently straighten your arms to push your body up and arch your back. Keep your legs and shoulders relaxed. Hold. Repeat a few times, as often as is comfortable.

SIDE GLIDE

LATERAL FLEXION

Stand with one shoulder leaning against a wall, feet together and slightly away from the wall and arms folded. Keeping your hips facing forward, let them slide toward the wall. Do not twist. Repeat a few times, then repeat on the other side
Note You may be advised to do this to one side only. Check with your physiotherapist or doctor.

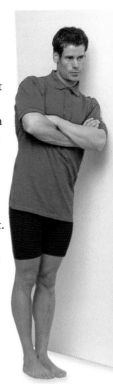

FORWARD DROP

ASSISTED FLEXION

Sit on a chair, with your hands clasped between your knees and your legs apart. Bend from your hips to drop your hands down to the floor and then slowly return to the upright position. Repeat.

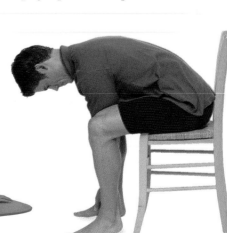

FORWARD LEAN

FLEXION & RELAXATION

1 Sit on a chair with your legs slightly apart and your feet raised on a step or some books. Clasp your hands together and, with your arms between your knees, lean forward.

2 Breathe in, pushing against the inside of your knees with your elbows. As you breathe out, stretch your arms down lower, feeling the stretch in your lower back.

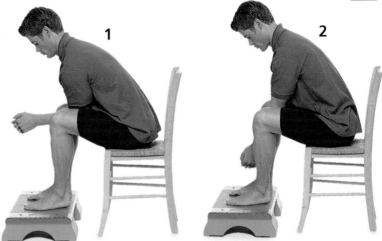

BODY CURL

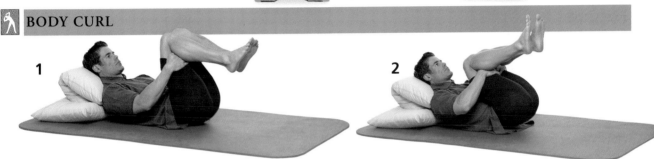

TRUNK FLEXION

Lie on your back on the floor with head and neck supported by pillows if this is more comfortable. Use your arms to draw both legs up to your chest (1). Hold the position as you breathe in and press your thighs outward, against your arms. As you relax and breathe out, let your knees come up further toward your chin (2). Repeat 2 to 3 times.

PELVIC STRETCH

ANTERIOR STRETCH

On your hands and knees, bend one knee and bring the leg up toward your body so that the foot is almost level with your hands. Stretch your other leg out behind you, with the knee straight. Breathe out as you push the straightened leg toward the floor and relax, feeling the stretch in the lower pelvic region.

Relax and repeat.

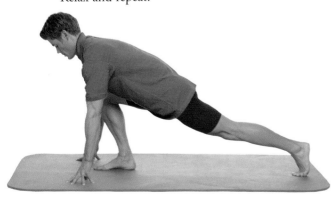

SIDE DROPS

SACRO-ILIAC MOBILITY

1 Kneel on one knee on the edge of a chair, so that your other knee drops down slightly lower than the seat.

2 Let that side of your body relax down toward the floor, then draw it up again. Keep your hips facing forward – don't tilt into or out from the chair. Repeat a few times, then turn and repeat on the other side.

Note You may be advised to do this to one side only. Check with your physiotherapist or doctor.

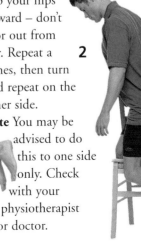

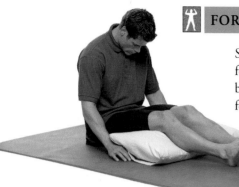

FORWARD SLUMP

Sit on the floor with a pillow under your knees. Gently bend forward so that your spine bends and stretches the lower back. Keep your arms relaxed by your sides. Hold for a few seconds and repeat 6 to 8 times.

KNEE BENDS

HIP EXTENSOR CONTROL

1 Lie on your front with your fingertips under your hip bones.
2 Keep abdominals tight as you slowly bend your knee. A "dip" of the pelvis – exerting pressure on your fingertips – indicates "give" in your back. If this occurs, start again, bending your leg very slowly and only as far as you can without feeling any change in pressure on your fingertips. Repeat with the other leg.
Note You may be advised to do this exercise with one leg only. Check with your physiotherapist or doctor.

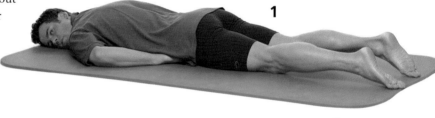

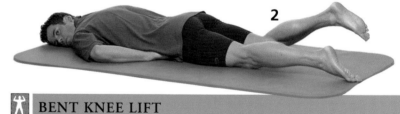

"THE WAITER'S BOW"

HIP FLEXION, STANDING

Stand behind a chair, with your feet slightly apart and your hands holding the back of the chair. Breathe out, bending at the hips so that your bottom sticks out and your back stays steady and relaxed. Hold and repeat.

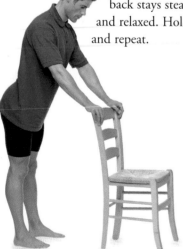

BENT KNEE LIFT

TRUNK STABILITY

Lie on your front with your fingertips under your "hip bones" and your leg bent at an angle of 90 degrees. Keep abdominals tight as you slowly lift your knee very slightly off the floor. A "dip" of the pelvis – exerting pressure on your fingertips – indicates "give" in your back. If this occurs, start again, bending your leg slowly and only as far as you can without feeling any change in pressure on your fingertips. Repeat with the other leg.
Note You may be advised to do this exercise with one leg only. Check with your physiotherapist or doctor.

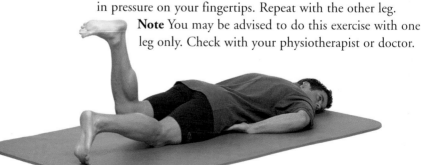

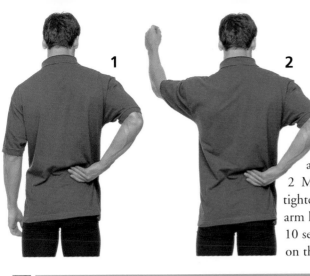

MUSCLE TONE

ERECTOR SPINAL MUSCLES

1 Standing, use the fingertips of one hand to feel the muscles on one side of the lower back, just below the waist and next to the spine.

2 Move your other arm up and down and notice how the muscles tighten. Practise making the muscles stay tight as you bring your arm lower. Aim to keep the muscles tight under your fingertips for 10 seconds. Work up to 10 repetitions of a 10-second hold. Repeat on the other side, as directed by your doctor or physiotherapist.

SUPINE CYCLING

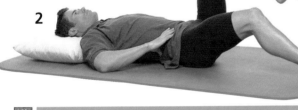

ABDOMINAL CONTROL

1 Lie on your back with your knees bent and your feet flat on the floor. Keep your abdominals taut as you gently lift both legs off the floor so that your thighs are vertical and your knees are bent at an angle of 90 degrees.

2 Gently lower one heel to the floor, slowly straightening that leg as far as you can without your back "giving".

3 Lift the leg back to the start position. Repeat, then repeat with the other leg, as directed by your physiotherapist.

LEG STRAIGHTENING

ABDOMINAL CONTROL

1 Lie on your back with your knees bent and your feet flat on the floor.

2 Keep your abdominals taut as you gently lift one foot off the floor and straighten that leg to its comfortable limit and as far as is possible without your back "giving". Once the leg is as straight as it will go, put your heel on the floor. Gently return to the starting position. Repeat. Then repeat the exercise with your other leg, as advised by your physiotherapist.

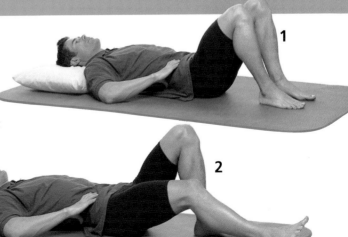

ADVANCED EXERCISES

Repeat all the strengthening exercises until fatigued, and the others as often as is comfortable – you should work up to the point of pain, but never beyond it. You physiotherapist may advise you to do any or all of these exercises on one side only.

FULL BACK STRETCH

SPINAL MOBILITY CONTROL

1 On your hands and knees, with your hands under your shoulders and arms straight, rock back to sit on your heels. Stretch your arms out and relax your head and neck.
2 Return to the hands-and-knees position and continue to move forward, bending your arms so that your lower back is arched and your stomach is on the floor. Return to the hands-and-knees position, leading with your bottom. Repeat.

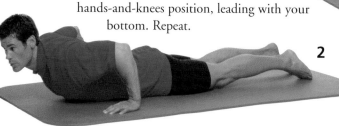

THIGH STRETCH

KNEE EXTENSION SITTING

Sit on a table with your legs relaxed and dangling down. Place your hands in the small of your back and use them to keep your back steady as you straighten your left leg as far as it can go without flexing your back. Your toes should point up. Repeat 3 to 4 times, then repeat with the other leg, as advised by your physiotherapist.

SPINAL MOBILITY

FLEXION EXTENSION & LATERAL FLEXION

Standing, lean forward, bending through the spine (1). Hold for 10 seconds. Reach down to one side, making sure that you do not twist your body – keep it facing forward (2). Hold. Stretch down to the other side (3). Hold. Lean back, using your hands on your lower back for support and to identify any stiff areas (4). Hold, then repeat the whole sequence.

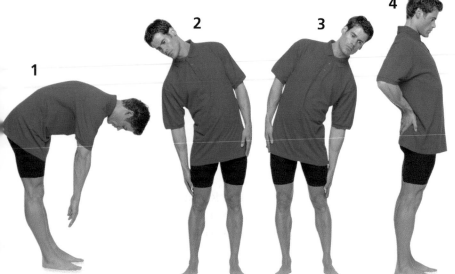

FORWARD STRETCH

ANTERIOR STRETCH

1 Lie on a table, with your legs dangling over the edge. Bend one leg up to your chest and hold it with your hands.
2 Lift your leg about 2.5 cm (1 inch). Hold for 2 seconds. Relax and let your lower leg drop down, feeling the stretch in the front of the thigh. Repeat 3 to 4 times, then repeat with your other leg.

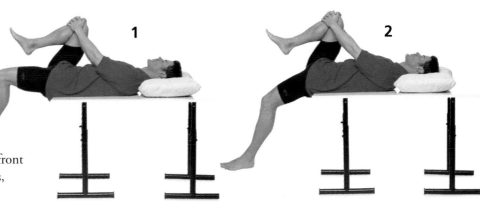

SIDE SCRUNCH

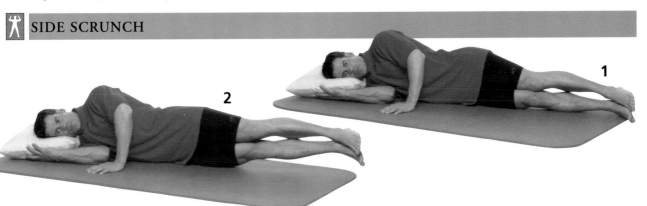

ABDOMINALS

1 Lie on your side with your head on a pillow and your legs out straight. Use your arm to support you as you lift both legs slightly off the floor. Remember to keep your legs in line with your body. Hold, relax and repeat, then repeat on the other side. **Note** You may be advised to do this exercise on one side only. Check with your physiotherapist.

ADVANCED SLUMP

Sit on the floor, with your legs straight out in front of you. Lean forward toward your toes, with your arms straight, your back slumping into a bend and your chin tucked in. Hold and feel the stretch in your lower back.

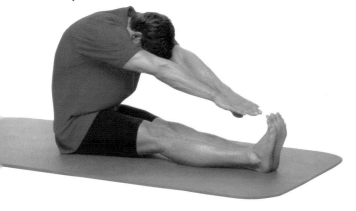

THIGH STRETCH

FEMORAL STRETCH

Standing, bend your leg up so that your foot comes up toward your buttock. Use your hand to pull the foot gently closer to your buttock to increase the stretch. Place your other hand on your stomach and use to it to ensure that your hips and stomach do not thrust forward. Keep your spine straight. Hold for 10 seconds. Repeat with the other leg as directed by your physiotherapist.

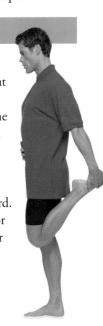

DOUBLE LEG LIFT

LOWER ABDOMINALS

1 Lie on your back with a pillow under your head if this is more comfortable. Bend your knees up toward your chest.
2 Using your hands flat on the floor to help you balance, contract your lower abdominal muscles to lift your bottom slightly off the floor. Repeat until fatigued.

DOUBLE LEG TWISTS

OBLIQUE ABDOMINALS

1 Lie on your back with a pillow under your head if this is more comfortable. Place a tennis ball between your knees and bend them up toward your chest.
2 Using your hands flat on the floor to help you balance, rotate your legs from side to side. Repeat until fatigued.

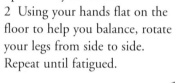

ADVANCED LEG LIFT

Lie on your back with a towel under your head and your legs straight. Keep your abdominals taut as you slowly draw your legs toward you, keeping your heels on the floor. Repeat and make sure that you can easily do 10 repetitions before you move on to lifting your legs up toward you with your heels raised up off the floor.

BACKWARD LEG LIFT

ERECTOR SPINAE

Stand next to a table with a pillow at its edge. Lie on the table so that your upper body is supported but your feet are still on the floor. Lift your legs, with your knees bent, so that your knees are no higher than the table. Repeat until fatigued. Variation: repeat the exercise with your ankles crossed.

MUSCLE TIGHTENING

ERECTOR SPINAE

Standing, use your fingertips to feel the muscles on one side of your lower back. Make the muscles tighten up under your fingertips. Hold the contraction for 10 seconds and repeat 10 times. Repeat on the other side.
Note You may be advised to do this exercise on one side only. Consult your doctor or physiotherapist.

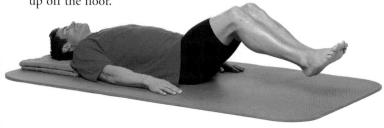

CURL DOWNS

ABDOMINAL CONTROL

1 Sit on the floor with your knees bent, feet flat on the floor and your arms by your sides.
2 Lower yourself gently toward the floor, keeping your back steady. Go as far as you can without your back "giving". Then gently lift yourself up and repeat. If you can curl down as far as the floor, use a towel to support your head. Repeat until fatigued.

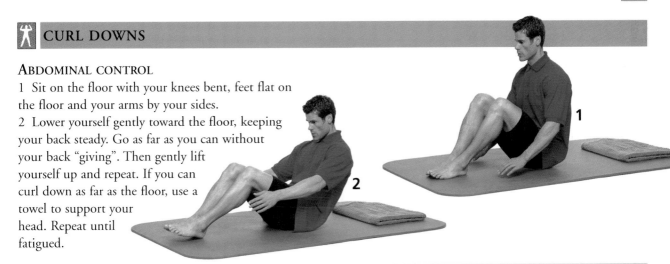

STRAIGHT LEG LIFT

EXTENSOR CONTROL

Lie on your front with your fingers under your "hip bones". Keep your abdominals taut as you gently lift one leg straight up from the floor. This is a small lift – the front of the thigh is raised just clear of the floor. Repeat until fatigued, alternating legs.
Note You may be advised to do this exercise on one side only. Consult your doctor or physiotherapist.

TWIST SIT-UPS

OBLIQUE ABDOMINALS

1 Lie on your back with your legs bent and your feet and knees slightly apart. Tighten your abdominals and interlink your fingers.
2 Leading with your hands, which should move across your body to the outside of one knee, raise your head and shoulders and twist your torso in a diagonal. Breathe out as you come up and in as you slowly roll back down, keeping the movement controlled.
3 Repeat to alternate sides until fatigued.

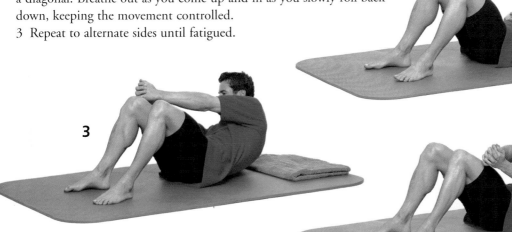

Gym Exercises

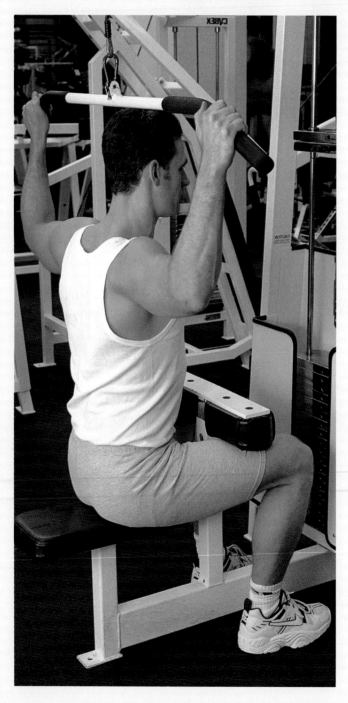

Generally speaking, most people are creatures of habit whose bodies will perform well those tasks which are required regularly. For instance, if you have three flights of stairs in your home and you use them regularly, you are unlikely to find the climb a problem. However, if you moved to a flat or bungalow, you would be making less demand on your leg muscles, heart and lungs. If, a month later, you tried climbing three flights of stairs several times in one day, you would feel it in your legs and you might also find yourself out of breath with your heart beating fast when you reached the top of the stairs.

AVOIDING INJURY IN SPORT

• Whatever your level of activity, your body can oblige if the demands on it are constant. If demand drops, your strength, flexibility and fitness will reduce. Similarly, if you increase demand too quickly, your tissues may not have time to adapt and this is when overuse injuries occur.

• Overuse injuries can occur at any age, but the older you get the more time the body will need to adapt to increased use.

• To confirm that an injury is due to overuse, look for changes in routine, an increase in frequency or vigour of exercise, or the introduction of a new activity.

• In the gym, overuse injuries occur because it is so easy to push yourself too hard – by increasing the resistance of the machine, increasing the number of repeats or simply going to the gym every day rather than once or twice a week.

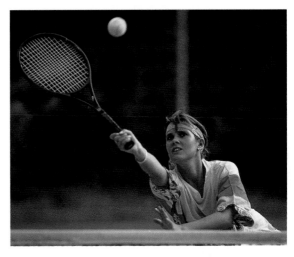

For tennis players overuse injuries are most common in the elbow, particularly if there is a change in the type of racquet, size of grip, frequency of play, surface on which they compete or general technique.

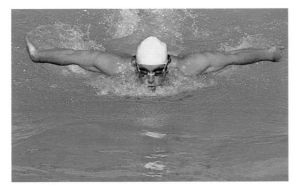

Swimmers risk overuse injury around the shoulders and upper back, particularly if they suddenly increase the distance they swim or the speed at which they do it. Always make any such changes gradually.

• The fact that you played a lot of sport years ago does not mean you are fit now, particularly if you drive to and from work and sit at a desk all day. You will need "warm-up exercises" to improve abdominal stability, hamstring flexibility and shoulder strength before you try lifting weights. Going straight from no exercise to working against resistance is inviting injury.

• This chapter shows some of the right and wrong ways of using gym equipment, as well as suggesting some exercises in this book which might help you to prepare yourself for a more strenuous routine.

WARMING UP

The following are a few suggested exercises for the warm-up part of your routine. Warming up is crucial because it eases the body gently into the work that you are about to ask it to do. It gets your cardiovascular system working efficiently – that is, it makes your heart pump blood round your body more vigorously, increasing the supply of oxygen to the muscles. Warming up also improves the spread of synovial fluid over the joint surfaces; its lubricating effect helps the joints move more freely and makes them less susceptible to injury.

Warm-up exercises should include smooth, rhythmic movements such as arm swinging (to loosen your shoulders) and gentle stretches. Repeat each exercise only as often as is comfortable. Ideally, some of the movements should imitate the exercise you are about to do – include gentle running on the spot if you are going running or jogging, for example. After 10 to 15 minutes, you should feel mildly exhilarated, your heart rate will have increased noticeably and you are ready to begin your full exercise routine. Other stretching exercises, for different parts of the body, can also be included at the end of your warm-up routine: try the Knee and Thigh Stretches on page 35; Hip and Hamstring Stretches on pages 43 and 52; Shoulder Stretches on pages 86–97 and Back Stretches on pages 114–115, 118–119, 124, 131, 135 and 138–141.

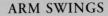

ARM SWINGS

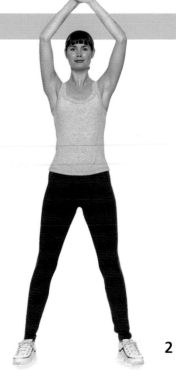

1 Start with your feet more than shoulder width apart and your knees bent. With your elbows slightly bent, cross your hands over in front of your body at about groin level. This should be a relaxed, comfortable position – do not tense your shoulders or legs.
2 Breathe in deeply. Holding that breath and straightening your legs, swing your arms out to your sides and up so that your hands cross over again above your head. Then breathe out as you swing your arms back down to the start position. Repeat without pausing 5 to 10 times.

1

2

STRETCHING

Breathe normally throughout this exercise and keep your back straight.
1 Stand up straight with your feet shoulder width apart, arms hanging loosely by your sides, knees slightly bent and stomach pulled in.
2 Slowly and gently raise your left arm to reach straight up above your head. At the same time, stretch your right arm down and out behind you as far as it will comfortably go. Hold for 1 to 2 seconds, then slowly return both arms to the starting position. Repeat the other way round, raising your right arm and stretching the left one out behind you. Repeat without pausing 5 to 10 times.

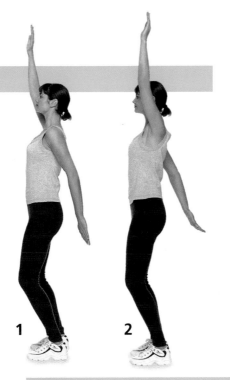

RUNNING

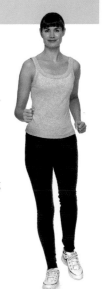

Run on the spot for 1 minute, lifting your knees as high as you can. Gradually increase the time to a maximum of 5 minutes. Try to land gently, letting your knees "give".

SKIPPING

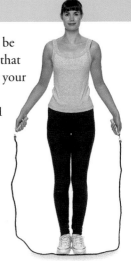

Choose a rope suitable for your height: it should be long enough not to trip you up, but not so long that there is lots of "spare" rope when you stand with your arms out at an angle of about 30 degrees.
Keeping your feet together, skip on the spot for 1 minute, rest and repeat. Do not jump up too high, and land gently, letting your knees "give". Gradually increase the time to a maximum of 5 minutes.
Variation: try "running skipping", leading with one foot for 1 minute, then with the other for 1 minute.

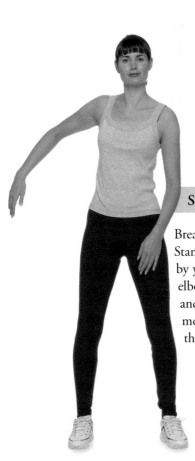

SHOULDER ROLLS

Breathe normally throughout this exercise and keep your back straight. Stand up straight with your feet shoulder width apart, arms hanging loosely by your sides, knees slightly bent and stomach pulled in. Bend your right elbow and lift your arm out to the side. Slowly rotate your shoulder up and forward, then down and back. Reverse the movement, so that you move your shoulder back first, then forward. Repeat with your left shoulder, then with both shoulders together. Repeat the whole sequence 5 to 10 times.

HAMSTRING CURL

This piece of equipment is a sort of arched bed on which you lie face down so that your bottom is higher than your head or feet. Your feet go under a movable bar, and the object is to bend your knees and lift this bar, exercising the hamstrings at the back of the thigh. The potential risk here is overextending the back.

WHAT TO DO

Lie face down, with your elbows bent and hands clasping the handles at the front of the bed. Tuck your ankles under the bar and bend your knees. Hold the position for a few seconds, feeling a stretch along the back of your thighs. Then lower the bar slowly and repeat in accordance with your normal programme. Keep your movements smooth and controlled. All the movement should come from your leg muscles. Hold the handles lightly for balance only – do not press down on them to help you lift.

Keep your head supported and your neck relaxed.

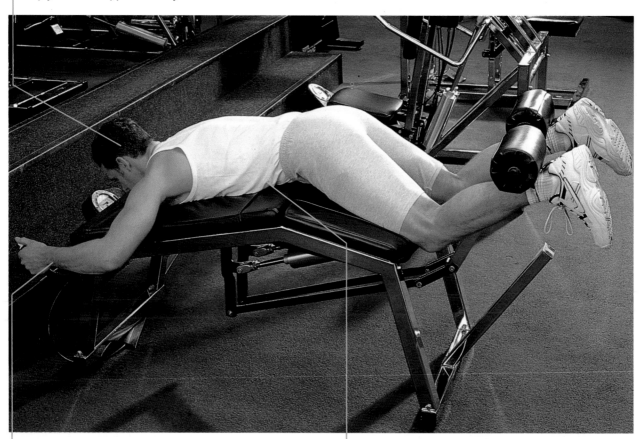

You should be lying comfortably before you start, with your back resting in a neutral position.

As you bend your knees, tighten your abdominals and squeeze your buttocks to stabilize your spine and pelvis.

WHAT NOT TO DO

If you are trying to lift too great a load or if you lack flexibility in your hamstrings, then as you work you will feel your back arching and hollowing in an effort to help the movement. This can cause back strain.

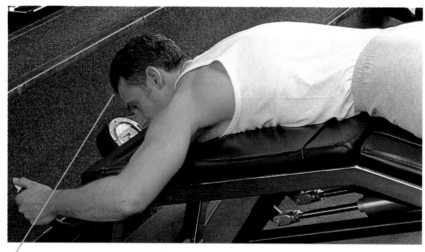

Do not raise your head – this puts unnecessary strain on the muscles of the neck and upper back.

As your legs straighten, make sure the front of your pelvis stays in contact with the table – this means that your back is steady.

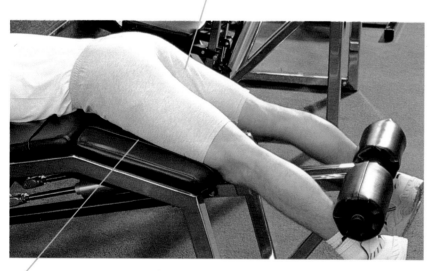

Do not use the muscles in your back to help you – all the movement should come from the hips and legs.

HELPFUL EXERCISES

Using the following exercises to complement your workout on the hamstring curl machine will help strengthen the muscles that the machine exercises and reduce the risk of injury.

PELVIC SQUEEZE
Beginners' hip exercise on page 45

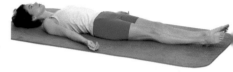

HAMSTRING LENGTHENING
Beginners' hip exercise on page 43

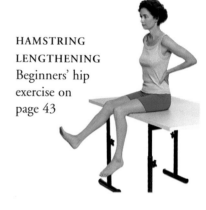

BENT KNEE LIFT
Intermediate lower back exercise on page 136

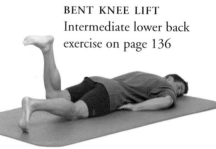

HEEL DRAG
Beginners' hip exercise on page 44

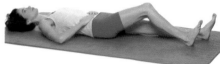

CYCLING MACHINE

The aim of the cycling machine is to strengthen the leg muscles and improve cardiovascular performance: it is excellent for the heart and lungs. Most cycling machines are adjustable, so that you can increase the resistance of the pedals, as if you were cycling uphill. Cycling is a useful warm-up exercise. Take it gently at first, with the machine on its lowest setting, and build up your speed gradually.

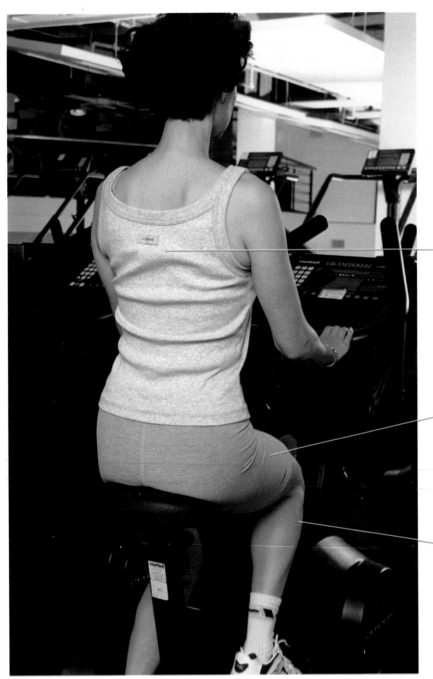

WHAT TO DO

● Before you begin, adjust the saddle to the right height. When your foot is at the lowest point on the pedal, your leg should be comfortably stretched, but the knee should not be locked.

● With a gym cycle you don't need to steer. Sit upright, either with your hands in your lap or with light pressure on the handlebars to help you balance.

● Pedal evenly and steadily, trying to put the same amount of pressure on each leg.

● Keep your knees over your toes.

WHAT NOT TO DO

If you lean too heavily on the handlebars, your neck and shoulders take unnecessary load; you lose the upright alignment of your spine. Pedalling too hard disturbs the alignment from your hips down through your knees.

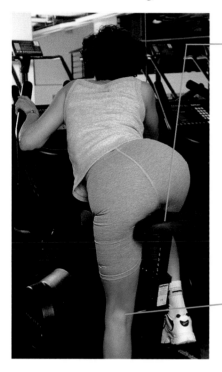

● Don't have the seat too high – if you stretch too far when you are pedalling, you will strain your lower back.

● Don't let your knees dip in toward your mid-line – this can lead to uneven wear on the kneecaps and pull on the iliotibial band along the outside of the thigh.

● WARNING
Stop immediately if you experience any of the following: chest pain, difficulty with breathing, faintness, severe aches and pains in the muscles or joints.

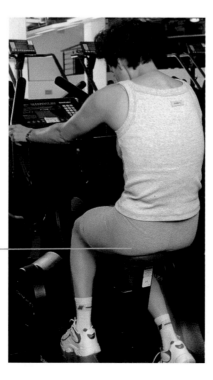

● Don't have the seat too low – this flexes the lower back, leading to strain and undue pressure on the intervertebral discs. It also makes your leg muscles work at an awkward angle.

HELPFUL EXERCISES

Try some of these exercises, taken from elsewhere in this book, before you use the cycling machine. They will help strengthen relevant parts of the body and make it less likely that you do yourself damage.

PRONE KNEE BEND
Intermediate hip exercise on page 48

HIP STRETCH
Intermediate hip exercise on page 46

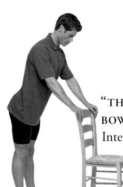

"THE WAITER'S BOW"
Intermediate lower back exercise on page 136

KNEE LOCK
Beginners' knee exercise on page 28

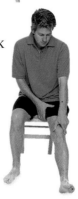

QUAD CURL

The purpose of this piece of equipment is to extend the legs and particularly strengthen the quadriceps, the large muscles at the front of the thigh.
Wrongly used, the machine can overextend the back or put strain on the knee joints and kneecaps.

WHAT TO DO

Sit comfortably in the chair with your knees bent and your feet tucked under the bar in front of you. Straighten your legs, pushing against the weight of the bar. Hold for a few seconds, control the bar as you lower it and repeat according to your normal exercise programme. Keep your movements smooth and controlled. All the movement should come from your leg muscles. Turning the lower leg in or out will put different emphasis on the inner and outer quadriceps muscles.

Keep your spine straight and your neck in line with it. Do not allow your head to jerk forward.

The bar should rest comfortably at the front of the ankle and can be adjusted.

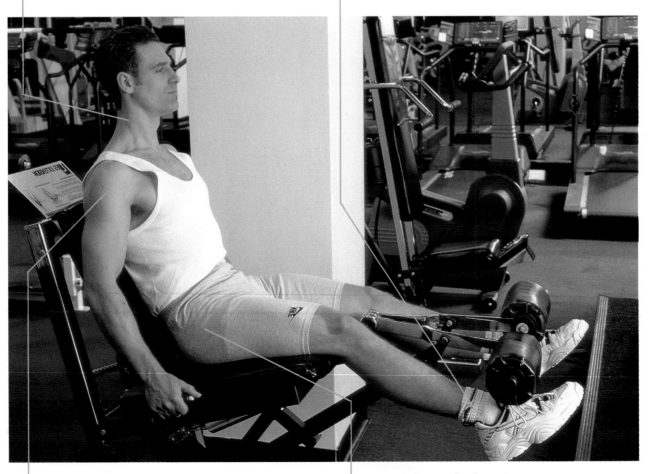

Do not tense your arms and shoulders – hold the handles lightly, for balance only.

Keep your bottom firmly on the seat.

WHAT NOT TO DO

Even with the machine at a low setting, this exercise can overwork your lower back if you lack flexibility. If you feel your back moving as your legs straighten, do not attempt to straighten them any further. It is better to work within a smaller range of movement until your flexibility improves.

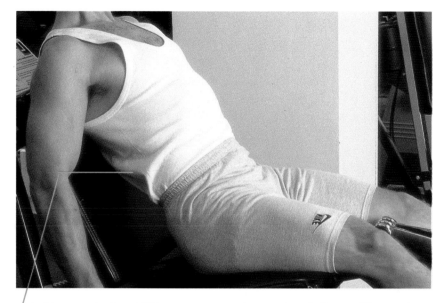

Arching your back and lifting your bottom off the seat as you push hard against the chair with your upper back and lower thighs may enable you to raise your legs further or lift a greater load, but it strains the spine and causes pain in the lower back.

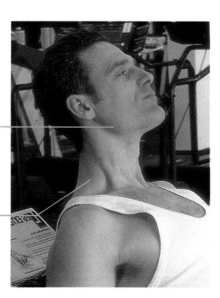

Do not stick your chin out – keep it tucked in to avoid overextending your neck.

Pushing too hard with the wrong muscles will strain the neck and shoulders.

HELPFUL EXERCISES

The following exercises, taken from earlier chapters in this book, will help you build up the muscles that you will be using on the quad curl machine.

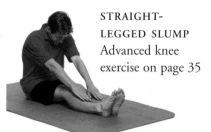

STRAIGHT-LEGGED SLUMP Advanced knee exercise on page 35

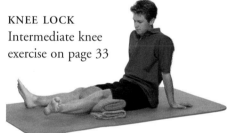

KNEE LOCK Intermediate knee exercise on page 33

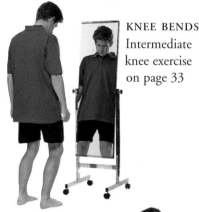

KNEE BENDS Intermediate knee exercise on page 33

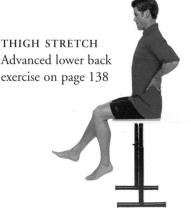

THIGH STRETCH Advanced lower back exercise on page 138

LAT PULL DOWN

At this machine, you sit holding an overhead crossbar, starting with your upper arms stretched out to the sides above shoulder level and your elbows bent. Pulling the crossbar down behind your head works the latissimus dorsi, the big delta-shaped muscle which reaches from the upper arm to the pelvis.

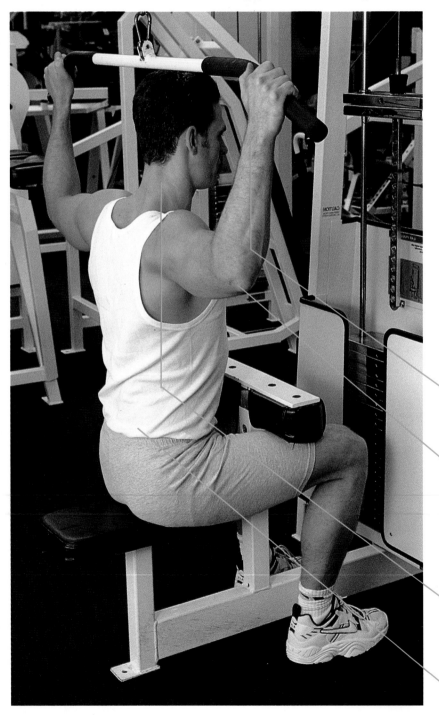

WHAT TO DO

Sit upright in the chair with your back and neck in line. A bar across your lap prevents you from lifting your knees and letting your thigh muscles do the work. Movement should come from your arms and shoulders. When the bar is at its highest point you should be able to grip it easily with your arms stretched up and elbows slightly bent. Pull the bar down until your hands are level with your shoulders, then control the bar as it returns to the starting position. Keep the movement smooth.

Move smoothly – do not jerk the bar up and down.

Keep your elbows out to your sides as your arms move down. If your elbows come forward, your shoulder joints will be "crammed" at the front.

Keep your upper back and neck as straight as possible throughout the movement.

Make sure your lower back remains upright.

WHAT NOT TO DO

If the latissimus dorsi is overworked, it can upset the balance of other muscles round the shoulders and neck. It can also become too tight and "throw out" your natural postural alignment.

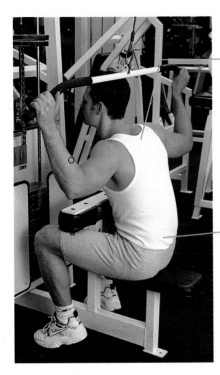

The commonest fault is poking your chin forward. This puts undue strain on the neck and upper back and could result in serious injury.

At the bottom of the movement, don't flex your back. This would mean you were bobbing up and down from the waist, rather than exercising the latissimus.

At the top of the movement, don't let your chin poke forward.

Don't try to stretch up too high – you will strain your shoulders and lower back.

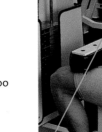

HELPFUL EXERCISES

These exercises will help build up the muscles you will be working on the lat pull down so that you do not hurt yourself by coming to it unprepared.

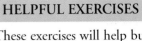

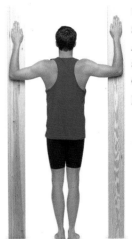

UPWARD STRETCH Advanced shoulder exercise on page 93

UPWARD STRETCH Advanced shoulder exercise on page 93

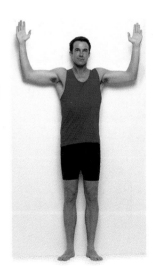

LONG STRETCH Advanced shoulder exercise on page 94

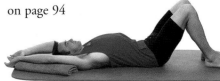

COOLING DOWN

It is every bit as important to spend 10 to 15 minutes "cooling down" at the end of your exercise session as it is to warm up. Do not neglect this part of the routine, however tired you are: just as you needed to raise the performance level of your cardiovascular system, so you now need to bring it gently back down to normal. If you stop exercising abruptly, blood may be trapped in the muscles, reducing blood supply to the rest of the body and leading to chest pains, dizziness and nausea. Excess lactic acid may build up round the joints, causing stiffness and reduced flexibility.

Any of the warm-up exercises given on pages 144–45 may be included in a cool-down programme. You might also like to try some of these.

KNEE LIFT AND TURN

1 Stand with your back straight, feet slightly apart, knees slightly bent and your stomach tucked in. Place your hands on your hips to help you balance – or use the back of a chair for support if this is easier. Gently raise your right knee until your thigh is parallel to the floor and your knee is bent at an angle of 90 degrees.
2 Slowly move your knee out to the right as far as it will comfortably go. Hold for 1 to 2 seconds, then bring your knee back to face forward and lower gently to the floor. Repeat using your left leg, then repeat the whole sequence 5 to 10 times.

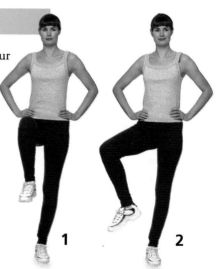

BEND AND SWING

1 Stand with your back straight, feet slightly apart, knees slightly bent and your stomach tucked in. Breathe in as you lift both arms to stretch out in front of you just above shoulder height.
2 Breathe out as you bend your knees and hips slowly and swing your arms straight out behind you just above your hips. Don't strain – take your arms just as far as is comfortable. Hold for 1 to 2 seconds, then breathe in and sweep your arms forward again, standing up as you do so to return to the start position. Keep your heels on the floor so that the straightening movement comes from your hips and knees. Repeat the whole sequence 5 to 10 times without pausing.

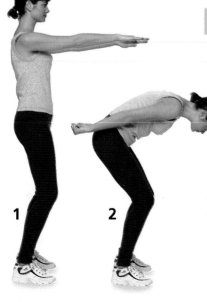

WAIST TWIST

1 Start in the same position as for the previous exercise. Lift your arms to stretch straight out in front of you at shoulder height.
2 Bend your right elbow and push it backward, twisting your upper body to the right as far as it will comfortably go. Do not move your hips – keep them facing forward. Hold the position for 1 to 2 seconds, then slowly turn to face the front again. Repeat on the other side, then repeat the whole sequence 5 to 10 times.

KNEE LIFT AND TURN

Stand with your back straight, feet slightly apart, knees slightly bent and your stomach tucked in. Without turning your hips, lift your right heel to your left buttock. Return slowly to the start position, then raise your left heel to your right buttock. If you can do this easily, add arm movements: swing your left arm back to touch your raised right foot, stretching your right arm out in front of you.

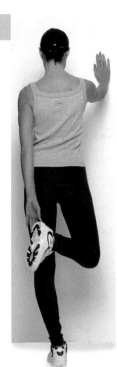

LUNGE

Start in the same position as for the Waist Twist, above. With your hands on your hips, breathe in and step forward with your left leg. Leave your right foot where it is. Holding your breath and keeping your back and neck straight, bend your left knee to an angle of about 90 degrees and drop your right knee toward the floor. When you begin to feel tension in your left knee, stop and hold that position for 8 to 10 seconds. Breathe out and gently lift yourself back to a standing position. Repeat with the right foot forward, then repeat the whole sequence 5 to 10 times.

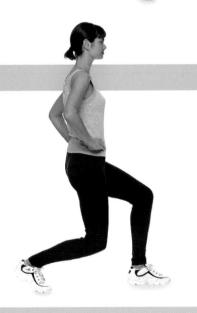

KNEELING STRETCH

1 Kneel on the floor, sitting on your heels with your arms stretched out in front of you, hands on the floor and back and neck straight. Gently push your arms forward as you lower your body closer to the floor. When you feel a stretch across your shoulders, stop and hold that position for 8 to 10 seconds. Slowly return to the start position and repeat 5 to 10 times.

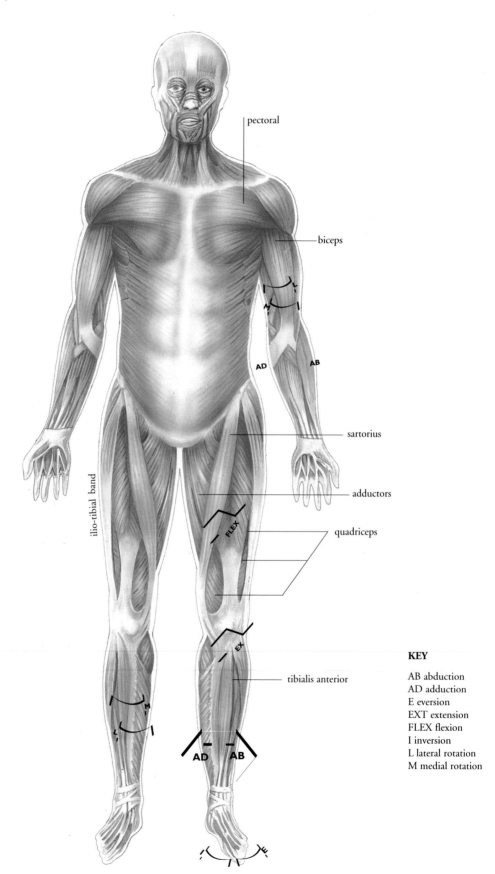

pectoral

biceps

AD

AB

sartorius

ilio-tibial band

adductors

FLEX

quadriceps

EX

tibialis anterior

M

L

I

AD AB

E

KEY

AB abduction
AD adduction
E eversion
EXT extension
FLEX flexion
I inversion
L lateral rotation
M medial rotation

GLOSSARY

The illustration shows the basic muscle and tendon structure of the human body and identifies the muscles, tendons and ligaments referred to in the text. It also illustrates the direction of the various movements given in the technical names for some exercises.

Collectively, muscles, tendons, ligaments and cartilage are known as "soft tissues". Voluntary muscles – those over which you exercise control – are attached to the skeleton and enable you to move and to stand upright. Tendons are a combination of fibrous and elastic tissue which connect the muscles to the bones. Ligaments run from one bone to another and support the joints. They are not as springy as tendons and may be injured by overstretching. In the early stages, a damaged ligament needs protection. Exercise should be gradually built up to allow the fibres to regain their supportive function. Cartilage is the slippery substance that covers bones at the joints and allows for friction-free movement.

It will help you plan your exercise routine if you understand the effect you are having on your soft tissues. Many of the flexibility and strength and stability exercises in this book indicate where you should feel the effect of what you are doing – this is one of the best ways of ensuring that you are doing the exercises correctly.

It is important to work on opposing muscle groups so that your body is balanced in terms of strength, stability and flexibility. For instance, strengthening the pectoral (chest) muscles can irritate the tissues round the shoulder if you do not balance the pectoral exercises with flexibility work and upper back strength. Similarly, building up the quadriceps (at the front of the thigh) can irritate the lower back if you do not balance your efforts with increased hamstring flexibility.

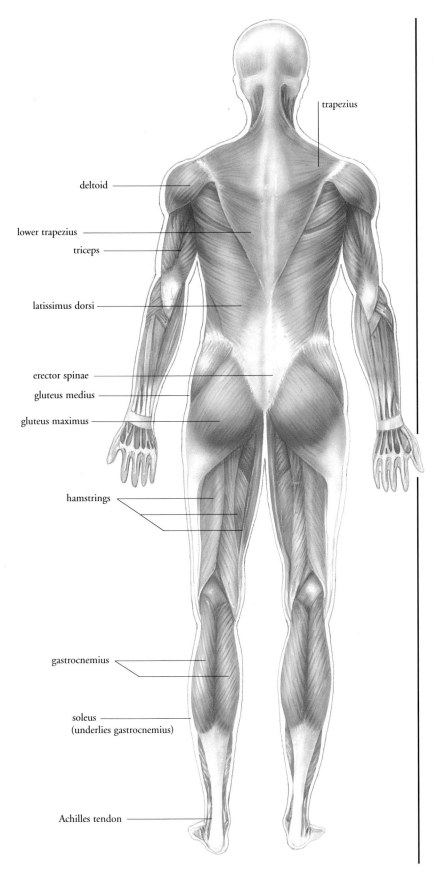

- trapezius
- deltoid
- lower trapezius
- triceps
- latissimus dorsi
- erector spinae
- gluteus medius
- gluteus maximus
- hamstrings
- gastrocnemius
- soleus (underlies gastrocnemius)
- Achilles tendon

INDEX

This index should be used in conjunction with the glosary (pages 156–7). Normal type indicates an entry in the text, **bold** indicates a major entry, and *italic* indicates that the information is contained in an illustration.

ACKNOWLEDGEMENTS

All photography by Andrew Sydenham except: wrist & hand (pages 56–69) by Henry Arden; gym equipment (pages 146–153) by Han Lee de Boer; page 143 top by Peter Grumann/The Image Bank; page 143 bottom by Michael K Daly/The Stock Market

Illustration (pages 156–157) by Mick Saunders
Gym facilities courtesy of Espree Health Club, London